The Healthy
Whole Body Reset for Seniors
Meal Plan

Carleigh Johnson

Contents

Introduction

Losing weight after 50 is a realistic goal. Maintaining a healthy weight can help you live an active and engaged life as a senior. However, many older people have to adjust their prior weight loss strategies to lose extra pounds safely. That's because what works for younger people when it comes to weight loss doesn't necessarily work for seniors.

But that doesn't mean you can't achieve your healthiest weight. You can lose weight as you get older by recognizing how your body changes with age and creating a safe, effective weight loss plan.

For many seniors, that process starts with determining their ideal weight. And because body composition changes with age, you may find that your goal weight and health priorities shift as you grow older. That's just one reason why it's essential to work closely with your healthcare team if you think that you need to lose weight.

This book will help you discover how to stay healthy while safely losing those extra pounds. So keep reading to learn more about how to create a sound plan for senior weight loss.

What Happens to our Body After 50?

The ways you take care of your body and how you stay active will dictate your quality of life and how good you will look. If you do not take care of your body, you might be fifty years old and look like you are sixty-five years old. But if you do good things for your body you might be sixty-five years old and look like you are fifty years old. Age is just a number. And even if you haven't been active in a long time, or ever, it is never too late to start on some sort of activity plan to increase the quality of your life.

I call it an activity plan because no one wants to exercise, right? So, let's think of this as an activity plan or a workout routine, both of those are positive statements that say you care about your body and want to fight the effects of growing older with everything you've got.

Once a person crosses that fifty-year mark, they begin losing one percent of their muscle each year. But muscle tone and fiber do not need to be lost with aging. With a proper workout, you can continue to build new muscle and maintain what you already have until you are in your nineties. And some of the exercises that you do for your muscles will help you build strong bones. This is especially important for women because losing the estrogen supplies in our bodies will cause us to lose bone mass faster than men. This is when we are really at risk for developing osteoporosis.

And regular physical activity will help you to avoid developing that middle-age spread around the abdomen or to lose it if you already have it. Activity will help you to maintain a proper weight for your height and build which in turn will help you to avoid many, if not all, of the age-related, obesity-related diseases such as cardiovascular diseases and diabetes.

Physical activity comes in four main types. Each one should be done at least once or twice a week to ensure your body is getting the right mix of activity.

The four main types of activity are:

Balance

Older people lose their sense of balance. It is easy for an older person to fall and break something, like a hip. When you engage in activities that help you to maintain your sense of balance will help reduce the risk that you might fall and suffer a permanent injury.

Stretching

As we age our muscles begin to lose their elasticity. This is part of why rolling out of bed in the morning gets more difficult as we get older.

Stretching activities will help you to improve and maintain your level of flexibility which will help you to avoid injuries to your joints and muscles.

Cardiovascular/Aerobic

These are also called endurance activities because you should be able to maintain them for at least ten minutes at a time. This key here is to get your heart working faster and your breathing to be deeper. You should be working hard but still able to carry on a conversation. These activities will strengthen your heart and lungs which are, after all, very important muscles in your body.

Strength training

We are not talking about bodybuilding, but if you want to go for it. This will include working out with resistance bands or lifting weights. Either activity will help to build muscle.

While there are four separate categories of exercise that does not mean that you need to keep them strictly separated because many activities will encompass work in more than one area. You can lift light weights while doing balance activities. Walking and swimming will build muscle strength and cardiovascular health. Yoga will improve balance and assist with building muscle strength and stretching. The key is to engage in seventy- five minutes of vigorous activity each week, or fifteen minutes five days each week; or you can get one hundred fifty minutes of moderate activity in five thirty-minute sessions each week.

And make sure that you design a plan that fits you. Remember that it is perfectly fine to change your routine as your needs change. Maybe, in the beginning, you will work on balance three days each week because you really need help with that. But after a few weeks, your balance has improved enough so that you can devote one of those days to strength training. This is your routine made just for you so make it work for you. And don't forget to get your doctor's okay before beginning any type of activity routine. He will most likely give you his blessings but it is always good to ask. He can also provide you with information on activities that are good for you personally.

One thing to note here, especially if you have not been active in a while, is not to begin a vigorous level of activity the same day you begin the keto diet. During the time your body is getting used to the diet and going through ketosis, you will not feel like indulging in a lot of extra activity and your workout routine will be doomed to failure. This journey is all about making you the best you possibly can so don't sabotage yourself in the first few weeks. If you really want to start your activities on day one of your diet then I recommend walking or bicycling. Either of these activities can be started slowly, so a gentle walk or bike around the neighborhood after dinner is a perfect activity.

Aging and Nutritional Needs

Nutrition is vital to maintain health and to lead an active and fulfilling life.

Childhood

In the initial years of life, the little bodies need essential nutrients along with natural nutrients to ensure they develop and grow physically and mentally. The food should provide high energy to support the rapid growth of bodies at this age. Also, childhood is the time of learning and experiencing new foods and developing taste and smell sense, which shape their eating habits for later in life. Therefore, children should be encouraged to consume a variety of foods every day. The key nutrient in children diet includes protein which is necessary for growth, calcium, and vitamin D to grow strong bones.

Adolescence

The body around this time goes through significant emotional and physical changes due to puberty. Moreover, maturing sexuality increases muscle growth and strengthens the bones, and this is a perfect opportunity for children to build strong bones for later. For this reason, the body must meet its calcium requirement. For this, dairy milk products are perfect healthy choices such as yogurt, milk, and cheese that are well known for high- quality protein and calcium-rich sources. Iron is also an essential bone nutrient that can be obtained from red meat, chicken, kidney beans, spinach, and mussels.

Teenage is also a time when children often tend to opt for junk foods and sugary drinks over more nutritious options. Encourage them to have water or milk as beverages and healthy snacks to combat craving and untimely hunger. Also, make-ahead some smoothies, prepare grab-and-go food options like toasts and sandwiches, and do meal prep for children that can't sit long enough to eat food at the meal table.

Adulthood

This is the time when you have to focus on maintaining the healthy body you have developed through your childhood and adolescence. Therefore, the body should get good enough nutrition like protein, calcium, vitamins, and phosphorus that helps you stay active, energetic, and maintain bones and muscles that tend to decrease as we move forward in age.

Older age

At the old age, the body needs the same or even more protein, minerals, and vitamins. For example, after the age of 50, your body's ability to absorb specific vitamins fades due to hormonal changes, and you don't have enough stomach acid to break down food sources. So, if you aren't eating foods that don't have these vitamins or not taking nutrients supplements, then you may suffer from dangerous ailments. In that case, eat little and often can effectively help your body in getting essential nutrients that support mobility, active mind, growth, mental and physical performance.

Enjoy a variety of foods and drinks and go for nutritious and natural options for foods that contain a range of nutrients. Similarly, you may not notice thirst in your later years, but keeping your body hydrated is important at any age.

Foods to Eat After 50

Once you are aware of the changes that you might experience at 50 and over, you should find out more about what nutrients your body needs and be sure to include them in your diet. Below I have listed some of the main nutrients that will be beneficial to your diet as you get older.

Protein

Protein is an important nutrient that your body needs to provide structure and maintenance to your cells and tissues and acts as a source of energy that your body can use to fuel itself throughout the day.

Protein can be found in animal products such as beef, chicken, eggs, fish, and tuna, as well as in almonds, broccoli, brussels sprouts, and dairy products like cottage cheese and plain Greek yogurt.

To calculate how much protein you should be consuming every day, you should first weigh yourself. For every kilogram of your body weight, it is recommended that you have a protein intake of 0.8 grams. Therefore, if you weigh 70 kilograms, then you should include 56 grams of protein per day in your diet.

Calcium

Calcium is another essential nutrient that you need in your diet that your body cannot produce on its own. It is especially important as you get older and experience bone loss. Calcium helps with a number of functions in your body, such as strengthening your teeth and bones and circulating blood and nutrients around your body.

You can find the best sources of calcium in dairy products such as cheese and plain Greek yogurt. However, if you are lactose intolerant or vegan, you will need to look at other sources of calcium, for example, calcium-fortified foods. Almonds, sardines, figs, and leafy greens like broccoli, kale, and spinach contain good sources of calcium, and you can include these in your diet.

A woman at the age of 50 should take 1,000 mg of calcium and 600 IU of vitamin D in their diet every day. Meanwhile, women over the age of 51 should increase their calcium intake to 1,200 mg, and women over the age of 70 should increase their daily vitamin D intake. You can take a calcium supplement if you are struggling to include the recommended amount in your diet.

Fiber

Fiber is a nutrient that helps to improve your metabolism, digest the food that you eat, keep your bowel movements regular, and lose weight, and keeps your blood sugar levels steady. Fiber can be a beneficial nutrient to consume in your diet and can assist in improving health conditions like diabetes.

Foods that are sources of fiber include all leafy greens, such as broccoli, brussels sprouts, and lettuce, as well as avocado, tomato, some berries, nuts like almonds and walnuts, and seeds like chia, flax, and hemp.

It is recommended that you include 25 grams of fiber every day in your diet. I suggest that you include a fiber supplement for the first few days if you are changing your diet to help you remain regular as your body gets used to the new foods.

Vitamin B12

Vitamin B12 is an essential nutrient that you should include in your diet. It helps to strengthen your brain function and keeps it from deteriorating as you get older, and it helps to produce oxygenated red blood cells that are transported through your body.

Vitamin B12 is found in animal products such as dairy, beef, chicken, eggs, and fish. If you are a vegetarian or vegan, vitamin B12 will be harder to include into your diet, but there are some fortified food alternatives, such as dairy, that you can use that have vitamin B12 added.

After 50, you have a greater risk of developing a vitamin B12 deficiency, which can be dangerous to your health. If there is concern that you are not receiving enough vitamin B12 in your diet, it is recommended that you consider taking a vitamin B12 supplement and including fortified food alternatives in your diet.

It is recommended that if you are over the age of 50 you should take 500 mcg of vitamin B12 each day and up to 1,000 mcg in more severe cases of deficiency.

Potassium

Potassium is a nutrient that you should include in your diet that helps your body to function properly by helping to improve digestion, stabilize your blood pressure, improve the signals that are transmitted along nerves in your body, and reduce your risk of osteoporosis and stroke. You can also use potassium as an electrolyte to replenish lost fluids in your body.

Foods that are sources of potassium include avocado, mushrooms, meat, salmon, almonds, hemp seeds, and leafy greens, such as broccoli, brussels sprouts, and spinach.

There is no specific amount of potassium that you are required to include in your diet, but it is suggested that you have s,500 mg each day to ensure that you don't develop a deficiency. You can include a potassium supplement if you are not consuming enough potassium in your diet.

Magnesium

Magnesium is another nutrient that you should include in your diet to ensure proper bodily functions. Magnesium helps with DNA synthesis, improves the signals that travel from your nerves to your brain, and stabilizes your blood pressure and blood sugar levels.

Foods that are sources of magnesium include almonds, avocados, spinach, and tofu.

It is recommended that a woman over the age of 50 should have s20 mg of magnesium each day. You can also include a magnesium supplement into your diet if you have a magnesium deficiency. One of the signs of a magnesium deficiency that I have noticed is that you might experience muscle cramps. By taking a magnesium supplement, you can reduce this occurrence.

Iron

Iron is an essential nutrient that your body needs so that oxygenated blood can be transported around your body.

Foods that are sources of iron include broccoli, spinach, tuna, shellfish, red meat, turkey, organ meats such as liver, kidneys, brain, and heart, as well as tofu and pumpkin seeds.

The amount of iron that you should have each day depends on various factors, such as your age, diet, genetics, and whether you are still menstruating or not. A woman who is 50 years old should take 18 mg of iron each day. However, if you are 51 and older, you will decrease your intake to 7 mg each day.

Omega-3 Fats

Omega-s fats are an essential nutrient that your body needs to help maintain and protect brain function and eyesight, and to improve your immune system against illnesses such as ADHD, breast cancer, and depression, as well as inflammatory diseases like arthritis.

Foods that contain omega-s fats include anchovies, chia seeds, cod liver oil, flax seeds, herring, mackerel, oysters, salmon, sardines, and walnuts.

If you are including fatty fish in your diet at least two times a week, then you should be meeting your omega-s dietary requirements. However, if you are not receiving enough omega-s in your diet, then it is recommended that you take an omega-s supplement.

Foods to Avoid After 50

These are the food you should avoid at 50.

Trans Fats

Fats that we receive from our diet can be grouped into three main categories: unsaturated fats, saturated fats, and trans fats. On the keto diet, you can use unsaturated and saturated fats in the meals that you eat and cook, but you should avoid using any trans fats.

When you include too many trans fats in your diet, such as baked goods, fried foods, hydrogenated vegetable oils, margarine, and ready-made meals, you increase your "bad" low-density lipoprotein (LDL) and decrease your "good" high-density lipoprotein (HDL).

When you consume trans fats, your body is unable to absorb these fats fully, and they accumulate in your blood and arteries. When this happens, your LDL cholesterol becomes elevated. LDL cholesterol can increase your blood pressure because your body has to work harder to pump blood through your body, and both of these factors can contribute to developing heart disease.

To decrease your LDL cholesterol levels, you should cut out trans fats from your diet and switch to healthy fats and oils that can increase your HDL cholesterol levels. HDL helps your body to decrease and protect against LDL cholesterol.

Although you can use saturated fats such as butter, cheese, and heavy cream in your diet, it is suggested that you try to limit them, as they can also elevate your cholesterol levels. Whenever possible, try to replace saturated and trans fats with healthy unsaturated fats, which include avocado, avocado oil, chia seeds, fatty fish, flax seeds, most nuts, olive oil, and olives.

Added Sugars

When you include too much sugar in your diet, triglyceride, which is the type of fat that is found in your bloodstream and tissues, is increased in your body. Your body then uses these triglycerides to provide you with energy when you are not receiving carbohydrates from foods—for example, between meals.

If your body is unable to burn this energy, your triglyceride levels will be elevated, which can cause your blood pressure and blood sugar levels to increase. When you continue to expose your body to high levels of triglycerides, you increase your risk of developing type 2 diabetes and heart disease.

When you choose to eat food that contains lots of sugar, your daily calorie intake will be high. If you do not burn off the extra calories in your diet from sugar and you are not active, you can gain weight. Excess weight can also be a contributing factor towards an increased risk in type 2 diabetes and heart disease.

To avoid picking up any additional weight as you turn 50 and older, you should limit the added sugars that you include in your diet and other food items that have a high sugar content. This includes chips, chocolate, desserts, pastries, soda, sweets, and food items that have sugar and sweeteners added to them, such as sweetened dairy products.

Sodium

Sodium is an important nutrient to include in your diet. The average adult aged 50 and older should receive 1,200 to 1,300 mg of sodium in their diet each day at minimum, but not more than 2,300 mg at most. The average American diet often sees people consuming as much as 3,400 mg of sodium each day, and this can be bad for your health.

Many people experience low blood pressure, and they need to include more sodium in their diet, while others experience high blood pressure and are advised to decrease their sodium intake. It is important that you find a balance between the minimum and maximum amounts that works for you and your diet to keep your sodium levels and blood pressure balanced throughout the day.

If you are including too much sodium in your diet, you should check the nutritional information of the foods you are eating and how much sodium they contain. Ready-made meals and processed foods contain high levels of sodium. We also tend to add extra salt and spices to our meals when we do not need to. To decrease your sodium intake, you should choose food options that contain less sodium in them and look at cutting down on how much salt and extra spices you add to your dishes.

Meal Planning and Its Benefits

Why people think meal planning is important might vary from person to person based on the what they value the most but no question most people see meal planning as a good practice that if done properly will have positive practical results but also aspirational benefits.

Why would you include another activity like meal planning in your to-dos list if you were not thinking of having positive results? after all we want to see the benefits of planning our meals, particularly when we keep realistic goals in mind.

Meal planning might seem structured, time-consuming or overdoing it but the reality is far from that.

On the contrary, meal planning is important because it helps you with the practical aspect of meal preparation from knowing what to cook, saving you money, reducing food waste and more.

No doubt both practical and aspirational aspects are important, so here we listed 12 reasons why meal planning is important:

Saves you money

Meal planning is a great way to save money on your food budget. People who plan their meals and cook at home could save between $10 to $15 per meal per person, which is equivalent to saving between $500 to $800 a year per meal per person.

By planning your meals you organize and control your grocery expenses avoiding buying more than what you need or even spending money on ingredients you will not use at all.

There are a few ways to approach your meal plan, for example, you can approach it by what you want to eat, how much time you want to spend in cooking, but also you can approach it by your weekly food budget. So, if shopping for groceries on a budget is important for you then meal planning is a must-try.

Saves you time

Meal planning is important because it helps you save time, you will even notice it at the first week of planning your meals.

When it comes to saving time, meal planning is a great tool, it helps you organize and being more efficient at time-consuming activities such as searching for recipes or creating grocery lists, not to mention the time you save by reducing the number of times you go to the shop.

Time saving is a direct result of having things organized upfront. The few minutes you take to plan your meals in advance will help you save hours during the week.

Reduce food waste

Meal planning plays an important role in helping you reduce food waste.

Food waste reduction is important for an overall positive impact but as well because it has a direct impact on your financials.

Food waste causes a big impact to our environment, and household food waste contributes to the problem. Of course we do not want to throw away food but most of the time we do it because lack of planning.

Meal planning helps you be more efficient at deciding the quantities of meals you and your family will consume, and this keeps you from throwing away food.

Makes it easy to improve cooking skills

Many people have different reasons to start meal planning, but no doubt that planning your meals is especially important when you are just starting cooking and your skills are not that good.

Improving cooking skills, as any other skill, is about practice, so you need to adopt a conscious but simple approach to go about it and planning your meal is the perfect way to do this. How? You could ask. Start at what you know best and expand from there.

For instance from knowing how to cook white rice, you could learn how to cook risottos. What about stir-fries? You could change the mix and change vegetables creating different meals, the point here is that you are using a cooking technique you are familiar and consciously choosing to cook different meals while improving your cooking skills.

Reduce stress

It's time to cook and you don't know what to prepare, or even worst you don't have the ingredients you need in your pantry or fridge but you need to put dinner on the table in the next hour. You are feeling frustrated and stressed.

Regardless whether you need to cook for your family or just for yourself, cooking, when you are not prepared, can be stressful. That is why meal planning is the favorite approach for many people who wants to have things organized and get rid of the stress that comes from not being ready.

You may think meal planning is too structured, but it does not have to be. It is a simple and a great way to organize meals, grocery lists and recipes and as a result you enjoy eating them with your family.

Helps with decision fatigue

Trying to come up with new healthy recipes every week can be daunting. Wouldn't it be great to have an approach to organize a list of meals you will cook during the next two weeks?

That approach exist, and it's called meal planning. Meal planning is a set-and-forget approach that is important to eliminate the decision fatigue of what to cook. Create a list of meals once a week or fortnightly, so you don't have to constantly decide what to have for dinner.

Helps you with aspirational diets

Meal planning is particularly important if you are about to start an aspirational diet, such as the Paleo diet.

To find common ingredients and cook healthy meals is sometime cumbersome as it is. Now imagine trying to do the same while following a specific diet and still providing food for your family. Now that calls for some planning.

Poor planning is the main reason we find it difficult to follow diets, and that includes having unrealistic goals.

So, if you want to have better chances to succeed in your diet then meal planning is the way to go because it helps you address realistic goals into specific actions, like identifying the meals you need to prepare, creating a calendar when you want to cook them, creating a grocery list, scheduling your grocery shopping, creating a list of favorite meals aligned with your diet.

Meal planning organise things for you upfront which helps you stick to your diet when willpower is not at its best.

Reduce risk of making poor food choices

We've been there before, a busy day left us with no time and energy and now it is time to cook. We just want to get it done, but with no idea of what to cook we "treat" ourselves with processed or fast food meal.

Whether because you feel tired or because you do not have time, making poor food choices can get into a bad habit and affect your health and the health of your family.

So how to avoid or reduce the risk of poor food choices? The key is planning. We know we'll have those situations where we'll not have the time and energy, so a simple strategy like meal planning is important to ensure you'll always have the ingredients you need to prepare healthy meals at home.

Reset Meal Plan

WEEK 1

MONDAY - DAY 1 – BREAKFAST

BACON & AVOCADO OMELET

Preparation Time: 5 minutes

Cooking Time: 5 minutes

Servings: 1

INGREDIENTS

1 slice crispy bacon

2 large organic eggs

5 cups freshly grated parmesan cheese

1 teaspoon finely chopped herbs

2 tablespoons ghee or coconut oil or butter

Half 1 small avocado

DIRECTIONS

1. Prepare the bacon to your liking and set aside. Combine the eggs, parmesan cheese, and your choice of finely chopped herbs. Warm a skillet and add the butter/ghee to melt using the medium-high heat setting. When the pan is hot, whisk and add the eggs.

2. Prepare the omelet, working it towards the middle of the pan for about 30 seconds. When firm, flip and cook it for another 30 seconds. Arrange the omelet on a plate and garnish with the crunched bacon bits. Serve with sliced avocado.

NUTRITION:

Calories: 719; Fat: 63g; Protein: 30g; Carbohydrates: 3.3g.

MONDAY - DAY 1 - LUNCH

BODY RESET GROUND BEEF AND GREEN BEANS

Preparation Time: 5 minutes

Cooking Time: 10 minutes

Servings: 2

INGREDIENTS

1 ½ ounce butter

8 ounces green beans, fresh, rinsed and trimmed

10 ounces ground beef

¼ cup crème fraîche or home-made mayonnaise, optional

Pepper and salt to taste

DIRECTIONS

1. Over moderate heat in a large, frying pan; heat a generous dollop of butter until completely melted.
2. Increase the heat to high and immediately brown the ground beef until almost done, for 5 minutes. Sprinkle with pepper and salt to taste.
3. Decrease the heat to medium; add more butter and continue to fry the beans in the same pan with the meat for 5 more minutes, stirring frequently.
4. Season the beans with pepper and salt as well. Serve with the leftover butter and add in the optional crème fraiche or mayonnaise, if desired.

NUTRITION:

Calories: 513; Fat: 44g; Protein: 30g; Carbohydrates: 8.5g.

MONDAY - DAY 1 - DINNER

PASTA FREE LASAGNA

Preparation Time: 20 minutes

Cooking Time: 56 minutes

Servings: 12

INGREDIENTS

2 large eggplants, cut into 1/8-inch thick slices lengthwise

Salt, as required

1 large organic egg

15 ounces part-skim ricotta

½ cup plus 2 tablespoons

Parmesan cheese, grated and divided

4 cups sugar-free tomato sauce

16 ounces part-skim mozzarella cheese, shredded

2 tablespoons fresh parsley, chopped

DIRECTIONS

1. Preheat the oven to 375°F.
2. Arrange the eggplant slices onto a smooth surface in a single layer and sprinkle with salt.
3. Set aside for about 10 minutes.
4. With a paper towel, pat dry the eggplant slices to remove the excess moisture and salt.
5. Heat a greased grill pan over medium heat and cook the eggplant slices for about 3 minutes per side.
6. Remove the eggplant slices from the grill pan and set aside.
7. In a medium bowl, place the egg, ricotta cheese and 1/2 cup of Parmesan cheese and mix well.
8. In the bottom of a 9x12-inch casserole dish, spread some tomato sauce evenly.
9. Place 5-6 eggplant slices on top of the sauce.

10. Spread some of the cheese mixture over eggplant slices and top with some of the mozzarella cheese.
11. Repeat the layers and sprinkle with the remaining Parmesan cheese.
12. Cover the casserole dish and bake for about 40 minutes.
13. Uncover the baking dish and bake for about 10 more minutes.
14. Remove the baking dish from oven and set aside for about 5-10 minutes before serving.
15. Cut into 12 equal-sized portions and serve, garnishing with fresh parsley.

NUTRITION

Calories: 200; Fat: 1g; Protein: 18.2g; Carbohydrates: 8g.

TUESDAY - DAY 2 - BREAKFAST
MORNING COCONUT PORRIDGE

Preparation Time: 1 minute

Cooking Time: 5 minutes

Servings: 1

INGREDIENTS:

1 egg, beaten

1 tablespoon coconut milk

2 tablespoons coconut flour

2 teaspoons butter

1 cup water

1 pinch salt

2 tablespoons flax seeds

Blueberries and raspberries

DIRECTIONS:

1. Put the flax seeds, coconut flour, water, and salt into a saucepan.
2. Heat this mixture until it has thickened slightly
3. Remove the mixture from the heat. Add beaten egg and put it on the stove again. Whisk slowly until you get a creamy texture.
4. Remove from the heat, add the butter and stir.
5. Serve with coconut milk, blueberries, and raspberries.

NUTRITION:

Calories 486; Fat 27g; Protein; 15g; Carbohydrates 6g.

TUESDAY - DAY 2 - LUNCH

CHEESY TILAPIA

Preparation Time: 10 minutes

Cooking Time: 10 minutes

Servings: 8

INGREDIENTS:

2 pounds tilapia fillets

½ cup Parmesan cheese, grated

3 tablespoons mayonnaise

¼ cup unsalted butter, softened

2 tablespoons fresh lemon juice

¼ teaspoon dried thyme, crushed

Salt and ground black pepper, to taste

DIRECTIONS:

1. Preheat the broiler of the oven.
2. Grease a broiler pan.
3. In a large bowl, mix together all ingredients except tilapia fillets. Set aside.
4. Place the fillets onto the prepared broiler pan in a single layer.
5. Broil the fillets for about 2-3 minutes.
6. Remove the broiler pan from the oven and top the fillets with cheese mixture evenly.
7. Broil for about 2 minutes further.
8. Serve hot.

NUTRITION:

Calories: 185; Fat: 9.8g; Protein: 23.2g; Carbohydrates: 1.4g.

TUESDAY - DAY 2 - DINNER

PAPRIKA CHICKEN

Preparation Time: 10 minutes

Cooking Time: 35 minutes

Servings: 4

INGREDIENTS:

4 chicken breasts, skinless and boneless, cut into chunks

2 tablespoons paprika

2 ½ tablespoons olive oil

1 ½ teaspoons garlic, minced

2 tablespoons fresh lemon juice

Pepper to taste

Salt to taste

DIRECTIONS:

1. Preheat the oven to 350°F.
2. In a small bowl, mix together garlic, lemon juice, paprika, and olive oil.
3. Season chicken with pepper and salt.
4. Spread 1/3 bowl mixture on the bottom of the casserole dish.
5. Add chicken into the casserole dish and rub with dish sauce.
6. Pour remaining sauce over chicken and rub well.
7. Bake for 30-35 minutes.
8. Serve and enjoy.

NUTRITION:

Calories: 380; Fat: 22g; Protein: 14g; Carbohydrates: 2.6g.

WEDNESDAY - DAY 3 - BREAKFAST

BREAKFAST ROLL-UPS

Preparation Time: 5 Minutes

Cooking Time: 15 Minutes

Servings: 5 roll-ups

INGREDIENTS:

Non-stick cooking spray

10 slices cooked bacon

1½ cups cheddar cheese, shredded

Pepper and salt

10 large eggs

DIRECTIONS:

1. Preheat a skillet on medium to high heat, then combine two of the eggs in a mixing bowl using a whisk.
2. After the pan has become hot, lower the heat to medium-low heat, then put in the eggs. If you want to, you can use some cooking spray.
3. Season eggs with some pepper and salt.
4. Cover the eggs and leave them to cook for a couple of minutes or until the eggs are almost cooked.
5. Drizzle around 1/3 cup of cheese on top of the eggs, then place 2 strips of bacon.
6. Roll the egg carefully on top of the fillings. The roll-up will almost look like a taquito. If you have a hard time folding over the egg, use a spatula to keep the egg intact until the egg has molded into a roll-up.
7. Put aside the roll-up, then repeat the above steps until you have four more roll-ups; you should have 5 roll-ups in total.

NUTRITION:

Calories: 412.2; Fat: 31.66g; Protein: 28,21g; Carbohydrates: 2.26g.

WEDNESDAY - DAY 3 – LUNCH

CAULIFLOWER AND CASHEW NUT SALAD

Preparation Time: 10 Minutes

Cooking Time: 5 Minutes

Servings: 4

INGREDIENTS:

1 head cauliflower, cut into florets

½ cup black olives, pitted and chopped

1 cup roasted bell peppers, chopped

1 red onion, sliced

½ cup cashew nuts

Chopped celery leaves, for garnish

For the dressing:

Olive oil Mustard Vinegar

Salt and pepper

DIRECTIONS:

1. Add the cauliflower into a pot of boiling salted water. Allow to boil for 4 to 5 minutes until fork-tender but still crisp.
2. Remove from the heat and drain on paper towels, then transfer the cauliflower to a bowl.
3. Add the olives, bell pepper, and red onion. Stir well.
4. Make the dressing: In a separate bowl, mix the olive oil, mustard, vinegar, salt, and pepper. Pour the dressing over the veggies and toss to combine.
5. Serve topped with cashew nuts and celery leaves.

NUTRITION:

Calories: 298; Fat: 20g; Protein: 8g; Carbohydrates: 4g.

WEDNESDAY - DAY 3 - DINNER
GARLICKY PRIME RIB ROAST

Preparation Time: 15 minutes

Cooking Time: 1 hour 35 minutes

Servings: 15

INGREDIENTS:

10 garlic cloves

2 teaspoons dried thyme

2 tablespoons olive oil

Salt

Ground black pepper

1 grass-fed prime rib roast

DIRECTIONS:

1. Mix the garlic, thyme, oil, salt, and black pepper. Marinate the rib roast with garlic mixture for 1 hour.
2. Warm-up oven to 500°F.
3. Roast for 20 minutes. Lower to 325°F and roast for 65-75 minutes.
4. Remove, then cool down for 10-15 minutes, slice, and serve.

NUTRITION:

Calories: 499; Fat: 25.9g; Protein: 61.5g; Carbohydrates: 0.7g.

THURSDAY - DAY 4 - BREAKFAST

BRACING GINGER SMOOTHIE

Preparation Time: 5 minutes

Cooking Time: 5 minutes.

Servings: 2

INGREDIENTS:

⅓ cup coconut cream

⅔ cup water

2 tablespoons lime juice

1 ounce spinach, frozen

2 tablespoons ginger, grated

DIRECTIONS:

1. Blend all the ingredients. Add 1 tablespoon lime at first and increase the amount if necessary.
2. Top with grated ginger and enjoy your smoothie!

NUTRITION:

Calories: 82; Fat: 8g; Protein: 1g; Carbohydrates: 3g.

THURSDAY - DAY 4 - LUNCH
CHICKEN AVOCADO SALAD

Preparation Time: 10 minutes

Cooking Time: 10 minutes

Servings: 3

INGREDIENTS:

2 chicken breasts, cooked and cubed

1 tablespoon fresh lime juice

2 avocados, peeled and pitted

2 Serrano chili peppers, chopped

¼ cup celery, chopped

1 onion, chopped

1 cup cilantro, chopped

1 teaspoon kosher salt

DIRECTIONS:

1. Scoop out the pulp from the avocados and place it in the bowl.
2. Mash the avocado flesh using a fork.
3. Add remaining ingredients and mix until well combined.
4. Serve and enjoy.

NUTRITION:

Calories: 236; Fat: 10.6g; Protein: 29g; Carbohydrates: 4.5g.

THURSDAY - DAY 4 - DINNER
EGG DROP SOUP

Preparation Time: 5 minutes

Cooking Time: 15 minutes

Servings: 2

INGREDIENTS:

3 cups chicken broth

2 cups Swiss chard chopped

2 eggs, whisked

1 teaspoon grated ginger

1 teaspoon ground oregano

2 tablespoons coconut aminos

Salt and pepper

DIRECTIONS:

1. Heat your broth in a saucepan.
2. Slowly drizzle in the eggs while stirring slowly.
3. Add the Swiss chard, grated ginger, oregano, and the coconut aminos. Next, season it and let it cook for 5-10 minutes.

NUTRITION:

Calories: 225; Fat: 19g; Protein: 11g; Carbohydrates: 4g.

FRIDAY - DAY 5 - BREAKFAST

BACON CHEESEBURGER WAFFLES

Preparation Time: 10 Minutes Cooking Time: 20 Minutes

Servings: 4

INGREDIENTS:

Toppings

Pepper and salt to taste

1 ½ ounces cheddar cheese

4 tablespoons sugar-free barbecue sauce

4 slices bacon

4 ounces ground beef, 70% lean meat and 30% Fat

Waffle dough

Pepper and salt to taste

3 tablespoons parmesan cheese, grated

4 tablespoons almond flour

¼ teaspoon onion powder

¼ teaspoon garlic powder

1 cup cauliflower crumbles

2 large eggs

1 ½ ounces cheddar cheese

DIRECTIONS:

1. Shred about 3 ounces of cheddar cheese, then add in cauliflower crumbles in a bowl and put in half of the cheddar cheese.
2. Put spices, almond flour, eggs, and parmesan cheese into the mixture, then mix and put aside for some time.
3. Thinly slice the bacon and cook in a skillet on medium to high heat.
4. After the bacon is partially cooked, put in the beef, cook until the mixture is well done.
5. Put the excess grease from the bacon mixture into the waffle mixture. Set aside the bacon mix.
6. Use an immersion blender to blend the waffle mix until it becomes a paste, then add half of the mix into the waffle iron and cook until it becomes crispy.
7. Repeat for the remaining waffle mixture.
8. As the waffles cook, add sugar-free barbecue sauce to the ground beef and bacon mixture in the skillet.
9. Then proceed to assemble waffles by topping them with half of the remaining cheddar cheese and half the beef mixture. Repeat this for the remaining waffles, broil for around 1-2 minutes until the cheese has melted, then serve right away.

NUTRITION:

Calories: 405; Fat: 33.9g; Protein: 18.8g; Carbohydrates: 4.4g.

FRIDAY - DAY 5 - LUNCH
SHRIMP STEW

Preparation Time: 15 minutes

Cooking Time: 20 minutes

Servings: 6

INGREDIENTS:

¼ cup olive oil

¼ cup onion, chopped

¼ cup roasted red pepper, chopped

1 garlic clove, minced

1 ½ pounds raw shrimp, peeled and deveined

1 (14-ounce) can sugar-free diced tomatoes with chilies

1 cup unsweetened coconut milk

2 tablespoons Sriracha

2 tablespoons fresh lime juice

Salt and ground black pepper, to taste

¼ cup fresh cilantro, chopped

DIRECTIONS:

1. In a wok, heat the oil over medium heat and sauté the onion for about 4–5 minutes.
2. Add the red pepper and garlic and sauté for about 4–5 minutes.
3. Add the shrimp and tomatoes and cook for about 3–4 minutes.
4. Stir in the coconut milk and Sriracha and cook for about 4–5 minutes.
5. Stir in the lime juice, salt and black pepper and remove from the heat.
6. Garnish with cilantro and serve hot.

NUTRITION:

Calories: 289; Fat: 16g; Protein: 27.1g; Carbohydrates: 7g.

FRIDAY - DAY 5 - DINNER

BODY RESET RED CURRY

Preparation Time: 20 minutes

Cooking Time: 15-20 minutes

Servings: 6

INGREDIENTS:

1 cup broccoli florets

1 large handful of fresh spinach

4 tablespoons coconut oil

¼ medium onion

1 teaspoon garlic, minced

1 teaspoon fresh ginger, peeled and minced

2 teaspoons soy sauce

1 tablespoon red curry paste

½ cup coconut cream

DIRECTIONS:

1. Add half the coconut oil to a saucepan and heat over medium- high heat.
2. When the oil is hot, put the onion in the pan and sauté for 3-4 minutes, until it is semi-translucent.
3. Sauté garlic, stirring, just until fragrant, about 30 seconds.
4. Lower the heat to medium-low and add broccoli florets. Sauté, stirring, for about 1-2 minutes.
5. Now, add the red curry paste. Sauté until the paste is fragrant, then mix everything.
6. Add the spinach on top of the vegetable mixture. When the spinach begins to wilt, add the coconut cream and stir.
7. Add the rest of the coconut oil, the soy sauce, and the minced ginger. Bring to a simmer for 5-10 minutes.
8. Serve hot.

NUTRITION:

Calories: 265; Fat: 7.1g; Protein: 4.4g; Carbohydrates: 2.1g.

SATURDAY - DAY 6 - BREAKFAST

SESAME BAGELS

Preparation Time: 10 minutes

Cooking Time: 15 minutes

Servings: 6

INGREDIENTS:

2 cups almond flour

3 eggs

1 tablespoon baking powder

2 ½ cups Mozzarella cheese, shredded

½ cream cheese, cubed

1 pinch salt

2-3 teaspoons sesame seeds

DIRECTIONS:

1. Preheat the oven to 425°F.
2. Use a medium bowl to whisk the almond flour and baking powder. Add the mozzarella cheese and cubed cream cheese into a large bowl, mix and microwave for 90 seconds. Place 2 eggs into the almond mixture and stir in thoroughly to form a dough.
3. Part your dough into 6 portions and make into balls. Press every dough ball slightly to make a hole in the center and put your ball on the baking mat.
4. Brush the top of every bagel with the remaining egg and top with sesame seeds.
5. Bake for about 15 minutes.

NUTRITION:

Calories: 469; Fat: 39g; Protein: 23g; Carbohydrates: 9g.

SATURDAY - DAY 6 - LUNCH

HEALTHY CELERY SOUP

Preparation Time: 10 minutes

Cooking Time: 20 minutes

Servings: 4

INGREDIENTS:

3 cups celery, chopped

1 cup vegetable broth

5 ounces cream cheese

1 ½ tablespoons fresh basil, chopped

¼ cup onion, chopped

1 tablespoon garlic, chopped

1 tablespoon olive oil

¼ teaspoon pepper

½ teaspoon salt

DIRECTIONS:

1. Heat some oil.
2. Add celery, onion and garlic to the saucepan and sauté for 4-5 minutes or until softened.
3. Add broth and bring to boil. Turn heat to low and simmer.
4. Add basil and cream cheese and stir until cheese is melted.
5. Season soup with pepper and salt.
6. Puree the soup until smooth.
7. Serve and enjoy.

NUTRITION:

Calories: 201; Fat: 5.4g; Protein: 5.1g; Carbohydrates: 3.9g.

SATURDAY - DAY 6 - DINNER

WINTER COMFORT STEW

Preparation Time: 15 minutes

Cooking Time: 50 minutes

Servings: 6

INGREDIENTS:

2 tablespoons olive oil

1 small yellow onion, chopped

2 garlic cloves, chopped

2 pounds grass-fed beef chuck, cut into 1-inch cubes

1 (14-ounce) can sugar-free crushed tomatoes

2 teaspoons ground allspice

1 ½ teaspoons red pepper flakes

½ cup homemade beef broth

6 ounces green olives, pitted

8 ounces fresh baby spinach

2 tablespoons fresh lemon juice

Salt and freshly ground black pepper, to taste

¼ fresh cilantro, chopped

DIRECTIONS:

1. In a pan, heat the oil over high heat and sauté the onion and garlic for about 2-3 minutes.
2. Add the beef and cook for about 3-4 minutes or until browned, stirring frequently.
3. Add the tomatoes, spices and broth and bring to a boil.
4. Reduce the heat to low and simmer, covered for about 30-40 minutes or until the desired doneness of the beef.
5. Stir in the olives and spinach and simmer for about 2-3 minutes.
6. Stir in the lemon juice, salt, and black pepper and remove from the heat.
7. Serve hot with the garnishing of cilantro.

NUTRITION:

Calories: 388; Fat: 17.7g; Protein: 48.5g; Carbohydrates: 8g.

SUNDAY - DAY 7 - BREAKFAST

MATCHA GREEN JUICE

Preparation Time: 10 minutes

Cooking Time: 0 minutes

Servings: 2

INGREDIENTS:

5 ounces fresh kale

2 ounces fresh arugula

¼ cup fresh parsley

4 celery stalks

1 (1-inch) piece fresh ginger, peeled

1 lemon, peeled

½ teaspoon matcha green tea

DIRECTIONS:

1. Add all ingredients into a juicer and extract the juice according to the manufacturer's method.
2. Pour into 2 glasses and serve immediately.

NUTRITION:

Calories: 113; Fat: 2.1g; Protein: 1.3g; Carbohydrates: 12.3g.

SUNDAY - DAY 7 - LUNCH

LEMONY SALMON

Preparation Time: 10 minutes

Cooking Time: 10 minutes

Servings: 4

INGREDIENTS:

1 tablespoon butter, melted

1 tablespoon fresh lemon juice

1 teaspoon Worcestershire sauce

1 teaspoon lemon zest, grated finely

4 (6-ounce) salmon fillets

Salt and ground black pepper, to taste

DIRECTIONS:

1. In a baking dish, place butter, lemon juice, Worcestershire sauce, and lemon zest, and mix well.
2. Coat the fillets with the mixture and then arrange skin side-up in the baking dish.
3. Set aside for about 15 minutes.
4. Preheat the broiler of the oven.
5. Arrange the oven rack about 6-inch from the heating element.
6. Line a broiler pan with a piece of foil.
7. Remove the salmon fillets from the baking dish and season with salt and black pepper.
8. Arrange the salmon fillets onto the prepared broiler pan, skin side down.
9. Broil for about 8-10 minutes.
10. Serve hot.

NUTRITION:

Calories: 253; Fat: 13.4g; Protein: 33.1g; Carbohydrates: 0.4g.

SUNDAY - DAY 7 - DINNER

YUMMY CHICKEN SKEWERS

Preparation Time: 10 minutes

Cooking Time: 10 minutes

Servings: 8

INGREDIENTS:

2 pounds chicken breast tenderloins

1 teaspoon lemon pepper seasoning

1 teaspoon garlic, minced

1 tablespoon olive oil

1 cup of salsa

DIRECTIONS:

1. Add chicken in a zip-lock bag along with 1/4 cup salsa, lemon pepper seasoning, garlic, and oil.
2. Seal bag and shake well and place it in the refrigerator overnight.
3. Thread marinated chicken onto the soaked wooden skewers.
4. Place skewers on hot grill and cooks for 8-10 minutes.
5. Brush with remaining salsa during the last 3 minutes of grilling.
6. Serve and enjoy.

NUTRITION:

Calories: 125; Fat: 2.5g; Protein: 24g; Carbohydrates: 2.1g.

WEEK 2

MONDAY - DAY 8 - BREAKFAST

COFFEE SURPRISE

Preparation Time: 5 minutes

Cooking Time: 5 minutes

Servings: 1 serving

INGREDIENTS:

2 heaped tablespoons flaxseed, ground

100ml cooking cream 35% Fat

½ teaspoon cocoa powder, dark and unsweetened

1 tablespoon goji berries

Freshly brewed coffee

DIRECTIONS:

1. Mix together the flaxseeds, cream and cocoa and coffee.

2. Season with goji berries.

3. Serve!

NUTRITION:

Calories: 55; Fat: 45g; Protein: 15g; Carbohydrates: 3g.

MONDAY - DAY 8 - LUNCH

BEEF SALAD WITH VEGETABLES

Preparation Time: 10 Minutes

Cooking Time: 10 Minutes

Servings: 4

INGREDIENTS:

1-pound (454 g) ground beef

¼ cup pork rinds, crushed

1 egg, whisked

1 onion, grated

1 tablespoon fresh parsley, chopped

½ teaspoon dried oregano

1 garlic clove, minced

Salt and black pepper, to taste

2 tablespoons olive oil, divided Salad:

1 cup chopped arugula

1 cucumber, sliced

1 cup cherry tomatoes, halved

1 ½ tablespoons lemon juice

Salt and pepper, to taste

DIRECTIONS:

1. Stir together the beef, pork rinds, whisked egg, onion, parsley, oregano, garlic, salt, and pepper in a large bowl until completely mixed.
2. Make the meatballs: On a lightly floured surface, using a cookie scoop to scoop out equal-sized amounts of the beef mixture and form into meatballs with your palm.
3. Heat 1 tablespoon olive oil in a large skillet over medium heat, fry the meatballs for about 4 minutes on each side until cooked through.
4. Remove from the heat and set aside on a plate to cool.
5. In a salad bowl, mix the arugula, cucumber, cherry tomatoes, 1 tablespoon olive oil, and lemon juice. Serve, season with salt and pepper.

NUTRITION:

Calories: 302; Fat: 13g; Protein: 7g; Carbohydrates: 6g.

MONDAY - DAY 8 - DINNER

CRAB-STUFFED AVOCADO

Preparation Time: 20 minutes

Cooking Time: 0 minutes

Servings: 2

INGREDIENTS:

1 avocado, peeled, halved lengthwise, and pitted

½ teaspoon freshly squeezed lemon juice

4 ½ ounces Dungeness crabmeat

½ cup cream cheese

¼ cup chopped red bell pepper

¼ cup chopped, peeled English cucumber

½ scallion, chopped

1 teaspoon chopped cilantro

Pinch sea salt

Freshly ground black pepper

DIRECTIONS:

1. Brush the cut edges of the avocado with the lemon juice and set the halves aside on a plate.
2. In a bowl or container, the crabmeat, cream cheese, red pepper, cucumber, scallion, cilantro, salt, and pepper must be well- mixed.
3. Divide the crab mixture between the avocado.
4. Serve and enjoy.

NUTRITION:

Calories: 239; Fat: 11.4g; Protein: 5.9g; Carbohydrates: 3.8g.

TUESDAY - DAY 9 - BREAKFAST

COCONUT PILLOW

Preparation Time: 10 minutes

Cooking Time: 0 minutes

Servings: 4 servings

INGREDIENTS:

1 can unsweetened coconut milk

Berries of choice

Dark chocolate

DIRECTIONS:

1. Refrigerate the coconut milk for 24 hours.
2. Remove it from your refrigerator and whip for 2-3 minutes.
3. Fold in the berries.
4. Season with the chocolate shavings.
5. Serve!

NUTRITION:

Calories: 50; Fat: 5g; Protein: 1g; Carbohydrates: 2g.

TUESDAY - DAY 9 - LUNCH

PARMESAN CHICKEN

Preparation Time: 10 minutes

Cooking Time: 35 minutes

Servings: 4

INGREDIENTS:

1 pound chicken breasts, skinless and boneless

½ cup parmesan cheese, grated

¾ cup mayonnaise

1 teaspoon garlic powder

½ teaspoon Italian seasoning

DIRECTIONS:

1. Preheat the oven to 375°F.
2. Spray baking dish with cooking spray.
3. In a small bowl, mix together mayonnaise, garlic powder, poultry seasoning, and pepper.
4. Place chicken breasts into the prepared baking dish.
5. Spread mayonnaise mixture over chicken then sprinkles cheese on top of chicken.
6. Bake chicken for 35 minutes.
7. Serve and enjoy.

NUTRITION:

Calories: 391; Fat: 23g; Protein: 16g; Carbohydrates: 11g.

TUESDAY - DAY 9 - DINNER

DELICIOUS TOMATO BASIL SOUP

Preparation Time: 10 minutes

Cooking Time: 40 minutes

Servings: 4

INGREDIENTS:

¼ cup olive oil

½ cup heavy cream

1 pound tomatoes, fresh

4 cups chicken broth, divided

4 cloves garlic, fresh

Sea salt and pepper to taste

DIRECTIONS:

1. Preheat oven to 400°F and line a baking sheet with foil.
2. Remove the cores from your tomatoes and place them on the baking sheet along with the cloves of garlic.
3. Drizzle the tomatoes and garlic with olive oil, salt, and pepper.
4. Roast at 400°F for 30 minutes.
5. Pull the tomatoes out of the oven and place into a blender, along with the juices that have dripped onto the pan during roasting.
6. Add two cups of the chicken broth to the blender.
7. Blend until smooth, then strain the mixture into a large saucepan or a pot.
8. While the pan is on the stove, whisk the remaining two cups of broth and the cream into the soup.
9. Simmer for about ten minutes.
10. Season to taste, then serve hot!

NUTRITION:

Calories: 225; Fat: 20g; Protein: 6.5g; Carbohydrates: 5.5g.

WEDNESDAY - DAY 10 - BREAKFAST

ALMOND COCONUT EGG WRAPS

Preparation Time: 5 minutes

Cooking Time: 5 minutes

Servings: 4

INGREDIENTS:

5 organic eggs

1 tablespoon coconut flour

2 ½ teaspoons sea salt

2 tablespoons almond meal

DIRECTIONS:

1. Combine the ingredients in a blender and work them until creamy. Heat a skillet using the med-high temperature setting.
2. Pour two tablespoons of batter into the skillet and cook - covered for about three minutes. Turnover and cook for another 3 minutes. Serve the wraps piping hot.

NUTRITION:

Calories: 111; Fat: 8g; Protein: 8g; Carbohydrates: 3g.

WEDNESDAY - DAY 10 - LUNCH

CREAMED SPINACH

Preparation Time: 10 minutes

Cooking Time: 15 minutes

Servings: 4

INGREDIENTS:

2 tablespoons unsalted butter

1 small yellow onion, chopped

1 cup cream cheese, softened

2 (10-ounce) packages frozen spinach, thawed and squeezed dry

2-3 tablespoons water

Salt and ground black pepper, as required

1 teaspoon fresh lemon juice

DIRECTIONS:

1. Melt some butter and sauté the onion for about 6–8 minutes.
2. Add the cream cheese and cook for about 2 minutes or until melted completely.
3. Stir in the water and spinach and cook for about 4–5 minutes.
4. Stir in the salt, black pepper, and lemon juice, and remove from heat.
5. Serve immediately.

NUTRITION:

Calories: 214; Fat: 9.5g; Protein: 4.2g; Carbohydrates: 2.1g.

WEDNESDAY - DAY 10 - DINNER

BEEF & MUSHROOM CHILI

Preparation Time: 15 minutes

Cooking Time: 3 hours 10 minutes

Servings: 8

INGREDIENTS:

2 pounds grass-fed ground beef

1 yellow onion

½ cup green bell pepper

½ cup carrot

4 ounces mushrooms

2 garlic cloves

1 can sugar-free tomato paste

2 tablespoons red chili powder

1 tablespoon ground cumin

1 teaspoon ground cinnamon

1 teaspoon red pepper flakes

½ teaspoon ground allspice

Salt

Ground black pepper

4 cups water

½ cup sour cream

DIRECTIONS:

1. Cook the beef for 8-10 minutes.
2. Stir in the remaining ingredient, except for the sour cream, and boil.
3. Cook on low, covered, for 3 hours.
4. Top with sour cream and serve.

NUTRITION:

Calories: 246; Fat: 15g; Protein: 25.1g; Carbohydrates: 8.2g.

THURSDAY - DAY 11 - BREAKFAST
BAGELS WITH CHEESE

Preparation Time: 10 minutes

Cooking Time: 15 minutes

Servings: 6

INGREDIENTS:

2 ½ cups Mozzarella cheese

1 teaspoon baking powder

3 ounces cream cheese

1 ½ cups almond flour

2 eggs

DIRECTIONS:

1. Shred the mozzarella and combine with the flour, baking powder, and cream cheese in a mixing container. Pop into the microwave for about one minute. Mix well.
2. Let the mixture cool and add the eggs. Break apart into six sections and shape into round bagels. Note: You can also sprinkle with a seasoning of your choice or pinch of salt if desired.
3. Bake them for approximately 12 to 15 minutes. Serve or cool and store.

NUTRITION:

Calories: 374; Fat: 31g; Protein: 19g; Carbohydrates: 8g.

THURSDAY - DAY 11 - LUNCH

PRAWNS SALAD WITH MIXED LETTUCE GREENS

Preparation Time: 10 Minutes

Cooking Time: 10 Minutes

Servings: 4

INGREDIENTS:

½ pound (227 g) prawns, peeled and deveined

Salt and chili pepper, to taste

1 tablespoon olive oil

2 cups mixed lettuce greens

For the dressing:

Mustard Aioli Lemon juice

DIRECTIONS:

1. In a bowl, add the prawns, salt, and chili pepper. Toss well.
2. Warm the olive oil over medium heat. Add the seasoned prawns and fry for about 6 to 8 minutes, stirring occasionally, or until the prawns are opaque.
3. Remove from the heat and set the prawns aside on a platter.
4. Make the dressing: In a small bowl, mix the mustard, aioli, and lemon juice until creamy and smooth.
5. Make the salad: In a separate bowl, add the mixed lettuce greens. Pour the dressing over the greens and toss to combine.
6. Divide the salad among four serving plates and serve it alongside the prawns.

NUTRITION:

Calories: 228; Fat: 17g; Protein: 5g; Carbohydrates: 3g.

THURSDAY - DAY 11 - DINNER
SPICED JALAPENO BITES WITH TOMATO

Preparation Time: 10 minutes

Cooking Time: 0 minutes

Servings: 4

INGREDIENTS:

1 cup turkey ham, chopped

¼ jalapeño pepper, minced

¼ cup mayonnaise

1/3 tablespoon Dijon mustard

4 tomatoes, sliced

Salt and black pepper, to taste

1 tablespoon parsley, chopped

DIRECTIONS:

1. In a bowl, mix the turkey ham, jalapeño pepper, mayo, mustard, salt, and pepper.
2. Spread out the tomato slices on four serving plates, then top each plate with a spoonful of turkey ham mixture.
3. Serve garnished with chopped parsley.

NUTRITION:

Calories: 250; Fat: 14.1g; Protein: 18.9g; Carbohydrates: 4.1g.

FRIDAY - DAY 12 - BREAKFAST
BACON & EGG BREAKFAST MUFFINS

Preparation Time: 15 minutes

Cooking Time: 30 minutes

Servings: 12

INGREDIENTS:

8 large eggs

8 slices bacon

2 green onions

DIRECTIONS:

1. Warm the oven at 350°F. Spritz the muffin tin wells using a cooking oil spray. Chop the onions and set aside.
2. Prepare a large skillet using the medium temperature setting. Fry the bacon until it's crispy and place on a layer of paper towels to drain the grease. Chop it into small pieces after it has cooled.
3. Whisk the eggs, bacon, and green onions, mixing well until all of the ingredients are incorporated. Place the egg mixture into the muffin tin (halfway full). Bake it for about 20 to 25 minutes. Cool slightly and serve.

NUTRITION:

Calories: 117; Fat: 8.6g; Protein: 8.9g; Carbohydrates: 0.6g.

FRIDAY - DAY 12 – LUNCH

MEATLESS CABBAGE ROLLS

Preparation Time: 25 minutes

Cooking Time: 25 minutes

Servings: 8

INGREDIENTS:

For Filling:

1 ½ cups fresh button mushrooms, chopped

3 ¼ cups zucchini, chopped

1 cup red bell pepper, seeded and chopped

1 cup green bell pepper, seeded and chopped

½ teaspoon dried thyme, crushed

½ teaspoon dried marjoram, crushed

½ teaspoon dried basil, crushed

Salt and freshly ground black pepper, to taste

½ cup homemade vegetable broth

2 teaspoon fresh lemon juice

For Rolls:

8 large cabbage leaves, rinsed

8 ounces sugar-free tomato sauce

3 tablespoons fresh basil leaves, chopped

DIRECTIONS:

1. Preheat the oven to 400°F. Lightly, grease a 13x9-inch casserole dish.
2. For filling: in a large pan, add all the ingredients except the lemon juice over medium heat and bring to a boil.
3. Reduce the heat to low and simmer, covered for about 5 minutes.
4. Remove from the heat and set aside for about 5 minutes.
5. Add the lemon juice and stir to combine.
6. Meanwhile, for rolls: in a large pan of boiling water, add the cabbage leaves and boil for about 2-4 minutes.
7. Drain the cabbage leaves well.
8. Carefully, pat dry each cabbage leaf with paper towels.
9. Arrange the cabbage leaves onto a smooth surface.
10. With a knife, make a V shape cut in each leaf by cutting the thick vein.
11. Carefully, overlap the cut ends of each leaf.
12. Place the filling mixture over each leaf evenly and fold in the sides.
13. Then, roll each leaf to seal the filling and secure each with a toothpick.

14. In the bottom of the prepared casserole dish, place 1/3 cup of the tomato sauce evenly.
15. Arrange the cabbage rolls over sauce in a single layer and top with remaining sauce evenly.
16. Cover the casserole dish and bake for about 15 minutes.
17. Remove from the oven and set aside, uncovered for about 5 minutes.
18. Serve warm, garnishing with basil.

NUTRITION:

Calories: 33; Fat: 0.4g; Protein: 2.2g; Carbohydrates: 8.5g.

FRIDAY - DAY 12 - DINNER
SPINACH & CHICKEN MEATBALLS

Preparation Time: 10 minutes

Cooking Time: 30 Minutes

Servings: 10

INGREDIENTS:

1 ½ pounds ground chicken

8 ounces Parmigiano-Reggiano cheese, grated

1 teaspoon garlic, minced

1 tablespoon Italian seasoning mix

1 egg, whisked

8 ounces spinach, chopped

½ teaspoon mustard seeds

Sea salt and ground black pepper, to taste

½ teaspoon paprika

DIRECTIONS:

1. Mix the ingredients until everything is well incorporated.
2. Now, shape the meat mixture into meatballs. Transfer your meatballs to a baking sheet and brush them with nonstick cooking oil.
3. Bake in the preheated oven at 350°F for about 25 minutes or until golden brown. Serve with cocktail sticks and enjoy!

NUTRITION:

Calories: 207; Fat: 12.3g; Protein: 19.5g; Carbohydrates: 4.6g.

SATURDAY - DAY 13 – BREAKFAST

KALE CHIPS

Preparation Time: 5 minutes

Cooking Time: 12 minutes

Servings: 2

INGREDIENTS:

1 bunch kale, removed from the stems

2 tablespoons extra virgin olive oil

1 tablespoon garlic salt

DIRECTIONS:

1. Preheat your oven to 350°F.
2. Coat the kale with olive oil.
3. Arrange on a baking sheet.
4. Bake for 12 minutes.
5. Sprinkle with garlic salt.

NUTRITION:

Calories: 100; Fat: 7g; Protein: 2.4g; Carbohydrates: 8.5g.

SATURDAY - DAY 13 - LUNCH
BODY RESET TACO SALAD

Preparation Time: 5 Minutes

Cooking Time: 20 Minutes

Servings: 4

INGREDIENTS:

1 pound ground beef

3 tablespoons olive oil

A dash of pepper

1 tablespoon onion powder

1 tablespoon cumin

1 tablespoon minced garlic clove

1 chopped tomato

½ cup sour cream

½ cup black olives

¼ cup cheddar cheese

2 tablespoons cilantro

1 chopped green pepper

DIRECTIONS:

1. With a taco salad, you will be able to enjoy everything that you love about tacos with a lot fewer carbohydrates! Whether you prepare this for taco Tuesday or a quick lunch, it is sure to be a crowd-pleaser!
2. Start this recipe by taking out your grilling pan and place it over a moderate temperature. As it warms up, you can add in the olive oil and let that sizzle. When you are set, add in the green pepper, spices, and ground beef. You can also use ground turkey in this recipe if that is more your style. Cook these ingredients together for ten minutes or so.
3. Next, place some mixed greens into a bowl and cover with the meat mixture you just created. If you would like some extra flavor, sprinkle some cheddar cheese over the top, along with some sour cream.

NUTRITION:

Calories: 138; Fat: 27g; Protein: 18g; Carbohydrates: 7g.

SATURDAY - DAY 13 - DINNER

ROASTED MACKEREL

Preparation Time: 10 minutes

Cooking Time: 20 minutes

Servings: 2

INGREDIENTS:

2 (7-ounce) mackerel fillets

1 tablespoon butter, melted

Salt and ground black pepper, to taste

DIRECTIONS:

1. Preheat the oven to 350°F.
2. Arrange a rack in the middle of the oven.
3. Lightly, grease a baking dish.
4. Brush the fish fillets with melted butter and then season with salt and black pepper.
5. Arrange the fish fillets into the prepared baking dish in a single layer.
6. Bake for about 20 minutes.
7. Serve hot.

NUTRITION:

Calories: 571; Fat: 41.1g; Protein: 47.4g; Carbohydrates: 7g.

SUNDAY - DAY 14 - BREAKFAST

HERBED COCONUT FLOUR BREAD

Preparation Time: 10 minutes

Cooking Time: 3 Minutes

Servings: 2

INGREDIENTS:

4 tablespoons coconut flour

½ teaspoon baking powder

½ teaspoon dried thyme

2 tablespoons whipping cream

2 eggs

Seasoning:

½ teaspoon oregano

2 tablespoons avocado oil

DIRECTIONS:

1. Take a medium bowl, place all the ingredients in it and then whisk until incorporated and smooth batter comes together.
2. Distribute the mixture evenly between two mugs and then microwave for a minute and 30 seconds until cooked.
3. When done, take out bread from the mugs, cut it into slices, and then serve.

NUTRITION:

Calories: 309; Fat: 26.1g; Protein: 9.3g; Carbohydrates: 5.3g.

SUNDAY - DAY 14 - LUNCH
MEXICAN PORK STEW

Preparation Time: 15 minutes

Cooking Time: 2 hours 10 minutes

Servings: 2

INGREDIENTS:

3 tablespoons unsalted butter

2 ½ pounds boneless pork ribs, cut into ¾-inch cubes

1 large yellow onion, chopped

4 garlic cloves, crushed

1 ½ cups homemade chicken broth

2 (10-ounce) cans sugar-free diced tomatoes

1 cup canned roasted poblano chiles

2 teaspoons dried oregano

1 teaspoon ground cumin

Salt, to taste

¼ cup fresh cilantro, chopped

2 tablespoons fresh lime juice

DIRECTIONS:

1. In a large pan, melt the butter over medium-high heat and cook the pork, onions, and garlic for about 5 minutes or until browned.
2. Add the broth and scrape up the browned bits.
3. Add the tomatoes, poblano chiles, oregano, cumin, and salt and bring to a boil.
4. Reduce the heat to medium-low and simmer, covered for about 2 hours.
5. Stir in the fresh cilantro and lime juice and remove from heat.
6. Serve hot.

NUTRITION:

Calories: 288; Fat: 10.1g; Protein: 39.6g; Carbohydrates: 8.8g.

SUNDAY - DAY 14 - DINNER

COLD GREEN BEANS AND AVOCADO SOUP

Preparation Time: 15 minutes

Cooking Time: 15 minutes

Servings: 4

INGREDIENTS:

1 tablespoon butter

2 tablespoon almond oil

1 garlic clove, minced

1 cup (227 g) green beans (fresh or frozen)

¼ avocado

1 cup heavy cream

½ cup grated cheddar cheese + extra for garnish

½ teaspoon coconut aminos

Salt to taste

DIRECTIONS:

1. Heat the butter and almond oil in a large skillet and sauté the garlic for 30 seconds.
2. Add the green beans and stir-fry for 10 minutes or until tender.
3. Add the mixture to a food processor and top with the avocado, heavy cream, cheddar cheese, coconut aminos, and salt.
4. Blend the ingredients until smooth.
5. Pour the soup into serving bowls, cover with plastic wraps and chill in the fridge for at least 2 hours.
6. Enjoy afterward with a garnish of grated white sharp cheddar cheese

NUTRITION:

Calories: 301; Fat: 3.1g; Protein: 3.1g; Carbohydrates: 2.8g.

WEEK 3

MONDAY - DAY 15 - BREAKFAST

BACON WRAPPED ASPARAGUS

Preparation Time: 10 minutes

Cooking Time: 20 minutes

Servings: 6

INGREDIENTS:

1 ½ pounds asparagus spears, sliced in half

6 slices bacon

2 tablespoons olive oil

Salt and pepper to taste

DIRECTIONS:

1. Preheat your oven to 400°F.
2. Wrap a handful of asparagus with bacon.
3. Secure with a toothpick.
4. Drizzle with the olive oil.
5. Season with salt and pepper.
6. Bake in the oven for 20 minutes or until bacon is crispy.

NUTRITION:

Calories: 166; Fat: 12.8g; Protein: 9.5g; Carbohydrates: 4.7g.

MONDAY - DAY 15 - LUNCH

CREAMY BROCCOLI AND LEEK SOUP

Preparation Time: 5 minutes

Cooking Time: 25 minutes

Servings: 4

INGREDIENTS:

10 ounces broccoli

1 leek

8 ounces cream cheese

3 ounces butter

3 cups water

1 garlic clove

½ cup fresh basil

Salt and pepper

DIRECTIONS:

1. Rinse the leek and chop both parts finely. Slice the broccoli thinly.
2. Place the veggies in a pot and cover with water and then season them. Boil the water until the broccoli softens.
3. Add the florets and garlic, while lowering the heat.
4. Add in the cheese, butter, pepper, and basil. Blend until desired consistency: if too thick, use water; if you want to make it thicker, use a little bit of heavy cream.

NUTRITION:

Calories: 451; Fat: 37g; Protein: 10g; Carbohydrates: 4g.

MONDAY - DAY 15 - DINNER

GARLIC BAKED BUTTER CHICKEN

Preparation Time: 10 minutes

Cooking Time: 40 minutes

Servings: 4

INGREDIENTS:

1 tablespoon rosemary leaves, fresh

3 chicken breasts, boneless, skinless (approximately 12 ounces); washed and cleaned

1 stick butter (½ cup)

½ cup Italian cheese, low Fat and shredded

6 garlic cloves, minced

Fresh ground pepper and salt to taste

DIRECTIONS:

1. Grease a large-sized baking dish lightly with a pat of butter, and preheat your oven to 375°F.
2. Season the chicken breasts with pepper and salt to taste; arrange them in the prepared baking dish, preferably in a single layer; set aside.
3. Now, over medium heat in a large skillet; heat the butter until melted, and then cook the garlic until lightly browned, for 4 to 5 minutes, stirring every now and then. Keep an eye on the garlic; don't burn it.
4. Add the rosemary; give everything a good stir; remove the skillet from heat.
5. Transfer the already prepared garlic butter over the meat.
6. Bake in the preheated oven for 30 minutes.
7. Sprinkle cheese on top and cook until the cheese is completely melted, for a couple of more minutes.
8. Remove from oven and let stand for a couple of minutes. Transfer the cooked meat to large serving plates. Serve and enjoy.

NUTRITION:

Calories: 375; Fat: 27g; Protein: 30g; Carbohydrates: 2.3g.

TUESDAY - DAY 16 - BREAKFAST

SHEET PAN EGGS WITH VEGGIES AND PARMESAN

Preparation Time: 5 minutes

Cooking Time: 15 minutes

Servings: 4

INGREDIENTS:

6 large eggs, whisked

Salt and pepper

1 small red pepper, diced

1 small yellow onion, chopped

½ cup diced mushrooms

½ cup diced zucchini

½ cup freshly grated parmesan cheese

DIRECTIONS:

1. Preheat the oven to 350°F and grease cooking spray on a rimmed baking sheet.
2. In a cup, whisk the eggs with salt and pepper until sparkling.
3. Add the peppers, onions, mushrooms, and courgettes until well mixed.
4. Pour the mixture into the baking sheet and scatter over a layer of evenness.
5. Sprinkle with parmesan, and bake until the egg is set for 13 to 16 minutes.
6. Let it cool down slightly, then cut to squares for serving.

NUTRITION:

Calories: 180; Fat: 10g; Protein: 14.5g; Carbohydrates: 5g.

TUESDAY - DAY 16 - LUNCH

STEAK WITH CHEESE SAUCE

Preparation Time: 15 minutes

Cooking Time: 17 minutes

Servings: 4

INGREDIENTS:

18 ounces grass-fed filet mignon

Salt

Ground black pepper

2 tablespoons butter

½ cup yellow onion

5 ¼ ounces blue cheese

1 cup heavy cream

1 garlic clove

Ground nutmeg

DIRECTIONS:

1. Cook onion for 5-8 minutes. Add the blue cheese, heavy cream, garlic, nutmeg, salt, and black pepper and stir.
2. Cook for about 3-5 minutes.
3. Put salt and black pepper in filet mignon steaks. Cook the steaks for 4 minutes per side.
4. Transfer and set aside. Top with cheese sauce, then serve.

NUTRITION:

Calories: 521; Fat: 22.1g; Protein: 44.7g; Carbohydrates: 3.3g.

TUESDAY - DAY 16 - DINNER
SCRUMPTIOUS CAULIFLOWER CASSEROLE

Preparation Time: 15 minutes

Cooking Time: 40 minutes

Servings: 4

INGREDIENTS:

1 large head cauliflower, cut into florets

2 tablespoons butter

2 ounces cream cheese, softened

1 ¼ cups sharp cheddar cheese, shredded and divided

1 cup heavy cream

Salt and freshly ground black pepper, to taste

¼ cup scallion, chopped and divided

DIRECTIONS:

1. Preheat the oven to 350°F.
2. In a large pan of boiling water, add the cauliflower florets and cook for about 2 minutes.
3. Drain cauliflower and keep aside.
4. For the cheese sauce: in a medium pan, add butter over medium-low heat and cook until just melted.
5. Add cream cheese, 1 cup cheddar cheese, heavy cream, salt and black pepper and cook until melted and smooth, stirring continuously.
6. Remove from heat and keep aside to cool slightly.
7. In a baking dish, place cauliflower florets, cheese sauce, and 3 tablespoons of scallion and stir to combine well.
8. Sprinkle with remaining cheddar cheese and scallion.
9. Bake for about 30 minutes.
10. Remove the casserole dish from oven and set aside for about 5-10 minutes before serving.
11. Cut into 4 equal-sized portions and serve.

NUTRITION:

Calories: 365; Fat: 33.6g; Protein: 12g; Carbohydrates: 5.6g.

WEDNESDAY - DAY 17 - BREAKFAST

CRISPY CHAI WAFFLES

Preparation Time: 10 minutes

Cooking Time: 20 minutes

Servings: 4

INGREDIENTS:

4 large eggs, separated into whites and yolks

3 tablespoons coconut flour

3 tablespoons powdered erythritol

1 ¼ teaspoon baking powder

1 teaspoon vanilla extract

½ teaspoon ground cinnamon

¼ teaspoon ground ginger

Pinch ground cloves

Pinch ground cardamom

3 tablespoons coconut oil, melted

3 tablespoons unsweetened almond milk Cocoa

DIRECTIONS:

1. Divide the eggs into two separate mixing bowls.
2. Whip the whites of the eggs until stiff peaks develop and then set aside.
3. Whisk the egg yolks into the other bowl with the coconut flour, erythritol, baking powder, cocoa, cinnamon, cardamom, and cloves.
4. Pour the melted coconut oil and the almond milk into the second bowl and whisk.
5. Fold softly in the whites of the egg until you have just combined.
6. Preheat waffle iron with cooking spray and grease.
7. Spoon into the iron for about 1/2 cup of batter.
8. Cook the waffle according to directions from the maker.
9. Move the waffle to a plate and repeat with the batter left over.

NUTRITION:

Calories: 215; Fat: 17g; Protein: 8g; Carbohydrates: 8g.

WEDNESDAY - DAY 17 - LUNCH
CREAMY KALE SALAD

Preparation Time: 15 minutes

Cooking Time: 0 minutes

Servings: 3

INGREDIENTS:

1 bunch spinach

1 ½ tablespoons lemon juice

1 cup sour cream

1 cup roasted macadamia

2 tablespoons sesame seeds oil

1 ½ garlic clove, minced

½ teaspoon black pepper

¼ teaspoon salt

2 tablespoons lime juice

1 bunch kale

Toppings

1 ½ avocado, diced

¼ cup pecans, chopped

DIRECTIONS:

1. Confirm that you have all the ingredients. Chop the kale, wash it, then remove the ribs.
2. Now transfer kale to a large bowl.
3. Add sour cream, lime juice, macadamia, sesame seeds oil, pepper, salt, garlic.
4. Finally, mix thoroughly. Top with your avocado and pecans. Serve and enjoy.

NUTRITION:

Calories: 291; Fat: 5.1g; Protein: 11.8g; Carbohydrates: 4.3g.

WEDNESDAY - DAY 17 - DINNER

SHRIMP CASSEROLE

Preparation Time: 15 minutes

Cooking Time: 30 minutes

Servings: 6

INGREDIENTS:

¼ cup unsalted butter

1 tablespoon garlic, minced

1 ½ pounds large shrimp, peeled and deveined

¾ teaspoon dried oregano, crushed

¼ teaspoon red pepper flakes, crushed

¼ cup fresh parsley, chopped

½ cup homemade chicken broth

1 tablespoon fresh lemon juice

1 (14½-ounce) can sugar-free diced tomatoes, drained

4 ounces feta cheese, crumbled

DIRECTIONS:

1. Preheat the oven to 350°F.
2. In a large wok, melt butter over medium-high heat and sauté the garlic for about 1 minute.
3. Add the shrimp, oregano and red pepper flakes and cook for about 4–5 minutes.
4. Stir in the parsley and salt and immediately transfer into a casserole dish evenly.
5. In the same wok, add broth and lemon juice over medium heat and simmer for about 2–3 minutes or until liquid reduces to half.
6. Stir in tomatoes and cook for about 2–3 minutes.
7. Pour the tomato mixture over shrimp mixture evenly and sprinkle with cheese.
8. Bake for approximately 15–20 minutes or until top becomes golden-brown.
9. Remove from the oven and serve hot.

NUTRITION:

Calories: 272; Fat: 13.9g; Protein: 29.8g; Carbohydrates: 6g.

THURSDAY - DAY 18 – BREAKFAST

LEMON & CUCUMBER JUICE

Preparation Time: 10 minutes

Cooking Time: 0 minutes

Servings: 2

INGREDIENTS:

2 large cucumbers, sliced

2 apples, cored and sliced

4 celery stalks

1 (1-inch) piece fresh ginger, peeled

1 lemon, peeled

DIRECTIONS:

1. Add all ingredients into a juicer and extract the juice according to the manufacturer's method.
2. Pour into 2 glasses and serve immediately.

NUTRITION:

Calories: 230; Fat: 2.1g; Protein: 1.2g; Carbohydrates: 1.3g.

THURSDAY - DAY 18 - LUNCH
VEGETABLE PATTIES

Preparation Time: 15 minutes

Cooking Time: 35 minutes

Servings: 4

INGREDIENTS:

1 tablespoon olive oil

1 onion, chopped

1 garlic clove, minced

1/2 head cauliflower, grated

1 carrot, shredded

3 tablespoons coconut flour

1/2 cup Gruyere cheese, shredded

1/2 cup Parmesan cheese, grated

2 eggs, beaten

1/2 teaspoon dried rosemary

Salt and black pepper, to taste

DIRECTIONS:

1. Cook onion and garlic in warm olive oil over medium heat, until soft, for about 3 minutes.
2. Stir in grated cauliflower and carrot and cook for a minute; allow cooling and set aside.
3. To the cooled vegetables, add the rest of the ingredients, form balls from the mixture, then press each ball to form a burger patty.
4. Set oven to 400°F and bake the burgers for 20 minutes.
5. Flip and bake for another 10 minutes or until the top becomes golden brown.

NUTRITION:

Calories: 315; Fat: 12.1g; Protein: 5.8g; Carbohydrates: 3.3g.

THURSDAY - DAY 18 - DINNER
CHICKEN ENCHILADA SOUP

Preparation Time: 10 minutes

Cooking Time: 45 minutes

Servings: 4

INGREDIENTS:

½ cup fresh cilantro, chopped

1 ¼ teaspoons chili powder

1 cup fresh tomatoes, diced

1 medium yellow onion, diced

1 small red bell pepper, diced

1 tablespoon cumin, ground

1 tablespoon extra-virgin olive oil

1 tablespoon lime juice, fresh

1 teaspoon dried oregano

2 cloves garlic, minced

2 large stalks celery, diced

4 cups chicken broth

8 ounces chicken thighs, boneless & skinless, shredded

8 ounces cream cheese, softened

DIRECTIONS:

1. In a pot over medium heat, warm olive oil.
2. Once hot, add celery, red pepper, onion, and garlic. Cook for about 3 minutes or until shiny.
3. Stir the tomatoes into the pot and let cook for another 2 minutes.
4. Add seasonings to the pot, stir in chicken broth and bring to a boil.
5. Once boiling, drop the heat to low and allow to simmer for 20 minutes.
6. Once simmered, add the cream cheese and allow the soup to return to a boil.
7. Drop the heat once again and let it simmer for another 20 minutes.
8. Stir the shredded chicken into the soup, along with the lime juice and the cilantro.
9. Spoon into bowls and serve hot!

NUTRITION:

Calories: 420; Fat: 29.5g; Protein: 27g; Carbohydrates: 12g.

FRIDAY - DAY 19 - BREAKFAST

CLASSIC WESTERN OMELET

Preparation Time: 5 minutes

Cooking Time: 10 minutes

Servings: 1

INGREDIENTS:

2 teaspoons coconut oil

3 large eggs, whisked

1 tablespoon heavy cream

Salt and pepper

¼ cup diced green pepper

¼ cup diced yellow onion

¼ cup diced ham

DIRECTIONS:

1. In a small bowl, whisk the eggs, heavy cream, salt, and pepper.
2. Heat up 1 teaspoon of coconut oil over medium heat in a small skillet.
3. Add the peppers and onions, then sauté the ham for 3 to 4 minutes.
4. Spoon the mixture in a cup, and heat the skillet with the remaining oil.
5. Pour in the whisked eggs and cook until the egg's bottom begins to set.
6. Tilt the pan and cook until almost set to spread the egg.
7. Spoon the ham and veggie mixture over half of the omelet and turn over.
8. Let cook the omelet until the eggs are set and then serve hot.

NUTRITION:

Calories: 415; Fat: 32.5g; Protein: 2.5g; Carbohydrates: 6.5g.

FRIDAY - DAY 19 - LUNCH

HERBED SALMON

Preparation Time: 10 minutes

Cooking Time: 8 minutes

Servings: 4

INGREDIENTS:

2 garlic cloves, minced

1 teaspoon dried oregano, crushed

1 teaspoon dried basil, crushed

Salt and ground black pepper, to taste

¼ cup olive oil

2 tablespoons fresh lemon juice

4 (4-ounce) salmon fillets

DIRECTIONS:

1. For salmon: In a large bowl, add all ingredients (except salmon) and mix well.
2. Add salmon and coat with marinade generously.
3. Cover and refrigerate to marinate for at least 1 hour.
4. Preheat the grill to medium-high heat. Grease the grill grate.
5. Place the salmon onto the grill and cook for about 4 minutes per side.
6. Serve hot.

NUTRITION:

Calories: 263; Fat: 19.7g; Protein: 22.2g; Carbohydrates: 0.9g.

FRIDAY - DAY 19 - DINNER

SPINACH AND ZUCCHINI LASAGNA

Preparation Time: 15 minutes

Cooking Time: 45 minutes

Servings: 4

INGREDIENTS:

2 zucchinis, sliced

Salt and black pepper to taste

2 cups ricotta cheese

2 cups shredded mozzarella cheese

3 cups tomato sauce

1 cup baby spinach

DIRECTIONS:

1. Let the oven heat to 375° and grease a baking dish with cooking spray.
2. Put the zucchini slices in a colander and sprinkle with salt.
3. Let sit and drain liquid for 5 minutes and pat dry with paper towels.
4. Mix the ricotta, mozzarella cheese, salt, and black pepper to evenly combine and spread 1/4 cup of the mixture in the bottom of the baking dish.
5. Layer 1/3 of the zucchini slices on top spread 1 cup of tomato sauce over, and scatter a 1/3 cup of spinach on top. Repeat process.
6. Grease one end of foil with cooking spray and cover the baking dish with the foil.
7. Let it bake for about 35 minutes. And bake further for 5 to 10 minutes or until the cheese has a nice golden-brown color.
8. Remove the dish, sit for 5 minutes, make slices of the lasagna, and serve warm.

NUTRITION:

Calories: 376; Fat: 14.1g; Protein: 9.5g; Carbohydrates: 2.1g.

SATURDAY - DAY 20 - BREAKFAST

FIVE GREENS SMOOTHIE

Preparation Time: 10 minutes

Cooking Time: 0 minutes

Servings: 3

INGREDIENTS:

6 kale leaves, chopped

3 celery stalks, chopped

1 ripe avocado, skinned, pitted, sliced

1 cup of ice cubes

2 cups spinach, chopped

1 large cucumber, peeled and chopped

Chia seeds to garnish

DIRECTIONS:

1. In a blender, add the kale, celery, avocado, and ice cubes, and blend for 45 seconds. Add the spinach and cucumber, and process for another 45 seconds until smooth.
2. Pour the smoothie into glasses, garnish with chia seeds, and serve the drink immediately.

NUTRITION:

Calories: 124; Fat: 7.8g; Protein: 3.2g; Carbohydrates: 3.5g.

SATURDAY - DAY 20 - LUNCH

OMELET-STUFFED PEPPERS

Preparation Time: 5 minutes

Cooking Time: 20 minutes

Servings: 2

INGREDIENTS

1 large green bell pepper, halved, cored

2 eggs

2 slices of bacon, chopped, cooked

2 tablespoons grated parmesan cheese

Seasoning:

1/3 teaspoon salt

¼ teaspoon ground black pepper

DIRECTIONS:

1. Turn on the oven, then set it to 400°F, and let preheat.
2. Then take a baking dish, pour in 1 tbsp. water, place bell pepper halved in it, cut-side up, and bake for 5 minutes.
3. Meanwhile, crack eggs in a bowl, add chopped bacon and cheese, season with salt and black pepper, and whisk until combined.
4. After 5 minutes of baking time, remove the baking dish from the oven, evenly fill the peppers with egg mixture and continue baking for 15 to 20 minutes until eggs have set.
5. Serve.

NUTRITION:

Calories: 428; Fat: 35.2g; Protein: 23.5g; Carbohydrates: 4.3g.

SATURDAY - DAY 20 - DINNER

WEEKEND DINNER STEW

Preparation Time: 15 minutes

Cooking Time: 55 minutes

Servings: 6

INGREDIENTS:

1 ½ pounds grass-fed beef stew meat, trimmed and cubed into 1-inch size

Salt and freshly ground black pepper, to taste

1 tablespoon olive oil

1 cup homemade tomato puree

4 cups homemade beef broth

2 cups zucchini, chopped

2 celery ribs, sliced

½ cup carrots, peeled and sliced

2 garlic cloves, minced

½ tablespoon dried thyme

1 teaspoon dried parsley

1 teaspoon dried rosemary

1 tablespoon paprika

1 teaspoon onion powder

1 teaspoon garlic powder

DIRECTIONS:

1. In a large bowl, add the beef cubes, salt, and black pepper and toss to coat well.
2. In a large pan, heat the oil over medium-high heat and cook the beef cubes for about 4-5 minutes or until browned.
3. Add the remaining ingredients and stir to combine.
4. Increase the heat to high and bring to a boil.
5. Reduce the heat to low and simmer, covered for about 40-50 minutes.
6. Stir in the salt and black pepper and remove from the heat.
7. Serve hot.

NUTRITION:

Calories: 293; Fat: 10.7g; Protein: 9.3g; Carbohydrates: 8g.

SUNDAY - DAY 21 - BREAKFAST

BACON & CHEESE FRITTATA

Preparation Time: 5 minutes

Cooking Time: 35 minutes

Servings: 6

INGREDIENTS:

1 cup heavy cream

6 eggs

5 crispy slices of bacon

2 chopped green onions

4 ounces cheddar cheese

DIRECTIONS:

1. Warm the oven temperature to reach 350°F.
2. Whisk the eggs and seasonings. Empty into the pie pan and top off with the remainder of the ingredients. Bake for 30-35 minutes. Wait for a few minutes before serving for best results.

NUTRITION:

Calories: 320; Fat: 29g; Protein: 13g; Carbohydrates: 2g.

SUNDAY - DAY 21 - LUNCH

LEMON ROSEMARY CHICKEN THIGHS

Preparation Time: 10 minutes

Cooking Time: 45 minutes

Servings: 4

INGREDIENTS:

4 chicken thighs, skinless

2 garlic cloves, roughly chopped

4 sprigs of Rosemary, fresh

1 lemon, medium

2 tablespoons butter

Pepper, and salt to taste

DIRECTIONS:

1. Preheat your oven to 400°F in advance and heat up a cast-iron skillet over high heat as well.
2. Season both sides of the meat with pepper, and salt. When the skillet is hot; carefully place the coated thighs, preferably skin side down into the hot skillet, and sear them for 4 to 5 minutes, until nicely brown.
3. Carefully flip and flavor the thighs with the lemon juice (only use ½ of the lemon). Quarter the leftover lemon halves and throw the pieces into the pan with the chicken.
4. Add the chopped garlic cloves together with some rosemary into the skillet.
5. Place the skillet inside the oven and bake for 30 minutes.
6. Remove the skillet from the oven. To add flavor, moisture, and more crispiness; add a portion of butter over the chicken thighs. Bake for 10 more minutes.
7. Serve hot and enjoy.

NUTRITION:

Calories: 159; Fat: 8.8g; Protein: 13.9g; Carbohydrates: 6.9g.

SUNDAY - DAY 21 - DINNER

NEW ENGLAND SALMON PIE

Preparation Time: 20 minutes

Cooking Time: 50 minutes

Servings: 5

INGREDIENTS:

For Crust:

¾ cup almond flour

4 tablespoons coconut flour

4 tablespoons sesame seeds

1 tablespoon psyllium husk powder

1 teaspoon organic baking powder

Pinch of salt

1 organic egg

3 tablespoons olive oil

4 tablespoons water

For Filling:

8 ounces salmon fillets

4 ¼ ounces cream cheese, softened

1 ¼ cups cheddar cheese, shredded

1 cup mayonnaise

3 organic eggs

2 tablespoons fresh dill, finely chopped

½ teaspoon onion powder

¼ teaspoon ground black pepper

DIRECTIONS:

1. Preheat the oven to 350°F. Line a 10-inch springform pan with parchment paper.

3. For crust: place all the ingredients in a food processor, fitted with a plastic pastry blade and pulse until a dough ball is formed.
4. Place the dough into prepared springform pan and with your fingers, gently press in the bottom.
5. Bake for about 12-15 minutes or until lightly browned.
6. Remove the pie crust from the oven and let it cool slightly.
7. Meanwhile, for filling: in a bowl add all the ingredients and mix well.
8. Place the cheese mixture over the pie crust evenly.
9. Bake for about 35 minutes or until the pie is golden brown.
10. Remove the pie from oven and let it cool slightly.
11. Cut into 5 equal-sized slices and serve warm.

NUTRITION:

Calories: 762; Fat: 70g; Protein: 24.8g; Carbohydrates: 10.8g.

WEEK 4

MONDAY - DAY 22 - BREAKFAST

ITALIAN-STYLE ASPARAGUS WITH CHEESE

Preparation Time: 10 minutes

Cooking Time: 10 Minutes

Servings: 2

INGREDIENTS:

½ pound asparagus spears, trimmed, cut into bite-sized pieces

1 teaspoon Italian spice blend

½ tablespoon lemon juice

1 tablespoon extra-virgin olive oil

4 tablespoons Romano cheese, freshly grated

DIRECTIONS:

1. Bring a saucepan of lightly salted water to a boil. Turn the heat to medium-low. Add the asparagus spears and cook for approximately 3 minutes. Drain and transfer to a serving bowl.
2. Add the Italian spice blend, lemon juice, and extra-virgin olive oil; toss until well coated.
3. Top with Romano cheese and serve immediately. Bon appétit!

NUTRITION:

Calories: 193; Fat: 14.1g; Protein: 11.5g; Carbohydrates: 5.6g.

MONDAY - DAY 22 - LUNCH

FRESH SUMMER SALAD

Preparation Time: 3 Minutes

Cooking Time: 0 Minutes

Servings: 4

INGREDIENTS:

2 tablespoons olive oil

1 tablespoon thyme

1 tablespoon oregano

¼ cup ricotta cheese

1 leaf, chopped basil

1 tablespoon balsamic vinegar

1 sliced cucumber

3 sliced tomatoes

5 sliced radishes

1 sliced onion

DIRECTIONS:

1. The first step for this recipe is to make your ricotta cheese. You can complete this in a small bowl by mixing the thyme, oregano, basil with the ricotta cheese.
2. Next, make your own dressing! For this task, whisk your vinegar and olive oil together. Once this is complete, season however you like.
3. Finally, take some time to slice and dice the vegetables according to the directions above. When your veggies are all set, assemble them in your serving dishes and pour the dressing generously over the top. As a final touch, dollop your ricotta cheese over your salad, and then your salad will be ready for serving.

NUTRITION:

Calories: 158; Fat: 19g; Protein: 16g; Carbohydrates: 4g.

MONDAY - DAY 22 - DINNER
MEATBALLS CURRY

Preparation Time: 15 minutes

Cooking Time: 25 minutes

Servings: 6

INGREDIENTS:

For Meatballs:

1 pound lean ground pork

2 organic eggs

3 tablespoons yellow onion

¼ cup fresh parsley leaves

¼ teaspoon fresh ginger

2 garlic cloves

1 jalapeño pepper

1 teaspoon Erythritol

1 tablespoon red curry paste

3 tablespoons olive oil

For Curry:

1 yellow onion

Salt

2 garlic cloves

¼ teaspoon ginger

2 tablespoons red curry paste

1 can unsweetened coconut milk

Ground black pepper

¼ cup fresh parsley

DIRECTIONS:

For meatballs:

1. Mix all the ingredients for the meatballs, except oil. Make small-sized balls from the mixture.
2. Cook meatballs for 3-5 minutes. Transfer and put aside.
   For curry:
3. Sauté onion and salt for 4-5 minutes. Add the garlic and ginger. Add the curry paste and sauté for 1-2 minutes. Add coconut milk, and meatballs, then simmer.
4. Simmer again for 10-12 minutes. Put salt and black pepper. Remove, then serve with fresh parsley.

NUTRITION:

Calories: 444; Fat: g; Protein: 17g; Carbohydrates: 8.6g.

TUESDAY - DAY 23 - BREAKFAST

BLT PARTY BITES

Preparation Time: 35 minutes

Cooking Time: 0 minute

Servings: 8

INGREDIENTS:

4 ounces bacon, chopped

3 tablespoons panko breadcrumbs

1 tablespoon Parmesan cheese, grated

1 teaspoon mayonnaise

1 teaspoon lemon juice

Salt to taste

½ heart Romaine lettuce, shredded

6 cocktail tomatoes

DIRECTIONS:

1. Put the bacon in a pan over medium heat.
2. Fry until crispy.
3. Transfer bacon to a plate lined with paper towel.
4. Add breadcrumbs and cook until crunchy.
5. Transfer breadcrumbs to another plate also lined with paper towel.
6. Sprinkle Parmesan cheese on top of the breadcrumbs.
7. Mix the mayonnaise, salt and lemon juice.
8. Toss the Romaine in the mayo mixture.
9. Slice each tomato on the bottom to create a flat surface so it can stand by itself.
10. Slice the top off as well.
11. Scoop out the insides of the tomatoes.
12. Stuff each tomato with the bacon, Parmesan, breadcrumbs and top with the lettuce.

NUTRITION:

Calories: 107; Fat: 6.5g; Protein: 6.5g; Carbohydrates: 5.4g.

TUESDAY - DAY 23 - LUNCH

GRILLED HALLOUMI CHEESE WITH EGGS

Preparation Time: 15 minutes

Cooking Time: 15 minutes

Servings: 4

INGREDIENTS:

4 slices Halloumi cheese

3 teaspoons olive oil

1 teaspoon dried Greek seasoning blend

1 tablespoon olive oil

6 eggs, beaten

½ teaspoon sea salt

¼ teaspoon crushed red pepper flakes

1 ½ cups avocado, pitted and sliced

1 cup grape tomatoes, halved

4 tablespoons pecans, chopped

DIRECTIONS:

1. Preheat your grill to medium.
2. Set the Halloumi in the center of a piece of heavy-duty foil.
3. Sprinkle oil over the Halloumi and apply the Greek seasoning blend.
4. Close the foil to create a packet.
5. Grill for about 15 minutes, then slice into four pieces.
6. In a frying pan, warm one tablespoon of oil and cook the eggs.
7. Stir well to create large and soft curds—season with salt and pepper.
8. Put the eggs and grilled cheese on a serving bowl.
9. Serve alongside tomatoes and avocado, decorated with chopped pecans.

NUTRITION:

Calories: 219; Fat: 5.1g; Protein: 3.9g; Carbohydrates: 1.5g.

TUESDAY - DAY 23 - DINNER

YELLOW CHICKEN SOUP

Preparation Time: 15 minutes

Cooking Time: 25 minutes

Servings: 5

INGREDIENTS:

2 ½ teaspoons ground turmeric

1 ½ teaspoons ground cumin

1/8 teaspoon cayenne pepper

2 tablespoons butter, divided

1 small yellow onion, chopped

2 cups cauliflower, chopped

2 cups broccoli, chopped

4 cups homemade chicken broth

1 ½ cups water

1 teaspoon fresh ginger root, grated

1 bay leaf

2 cups Swiss chard, stemmed and chopped finely

½ cup unsweetened coconut milk

3 (4-ounce) grass-fed boneless, skinless chicken thighs, cut into bite-size pieces

2 tablespoons fresh lime juice

DIRECTIONS:

1. In a small bowl, mix together the turmeric, cumin, and cayenne pepper and set aside.
2. In a large pan, melt 1 tablespoon of butter over medium heat and sauté the onion for about 3-4 minutes.
3. Add the cauliflower, broccoli, and half of the spice mixture and cook for another 3-4 minutes.
4. Add the broth, water, ginger, and bay leaf and bring to a boil.
5. Reduce the heat to low and simmer for about 8-10 minutes.
6. Stir in the Swiss chard and coconut milk and cook for about 1-2 minutes.
7. Meanwhile, in a large skillet, melt the remaining butter over medium heat and sear the chicken pieces for about 5 minutes.
8. Stir in the remaining spice mix and cook for about 5 minutes, stirring frequently.
9. Transfer the soup into serving bowls and top with the chicken pieces.
10. Drizzle with lime juice and serve.

NUTRITION:

Calories: 258; Fat: 16.8g; Protein: 18.4g; Carbohydrates: 8.4g.

WEDNESDAY - DAY 24 - BREAKFAST

ALMOND BUTTER MUFFINS

Preparation Time: 10 minutes

Cooking Time: 25 minutes

Servings: 6

INGREDIENTS:

1 cups almond flour

½ cup powdered erythritol

1 teaspoons baking powder

¼ teaspoon salt

¾ cup almond butter, warmed

¾ cup unsweetened almond milk

2 large eggs

DIRECTIONS:

1. Preheat the oven to 350°F, and line a paper liner muffin pan.
2. In a mixing bowl, whisk the almond flour and the erythritol, baking powder, and salt.
3. Whisk the almond milk, almond butter, and the eggs together in a separate bowl.
4. Drop the wet ingredients into the dry until just mixed together.
5. Spoon the batter into the prepared pan and bake for 22 to 25 minutes until clean comes out the knife inserted in the middle.
6. Let cool and enjoy.

NUTRITION:

Calories: 135; Fat: 11g; Protein: 6g; Carbohydrates: 4g.

WEDNESDAY - DAY 24 - LUNCH

GRILLED STEAK

Preparation Time: 15 minutes

Cooking Time: 12 minutes

Servings: 6

INGREDIENTS:

1 teaspoon lemon zest

1 garlic clove

1 tablespoon red chili powder

1 tablespoon paprika

1 tablespoon ground coffee

Salt

Ground black pepper

2 grass-fed skirt steaks

DIRECTIONS:

1. Mix all the ingredients except steaks. Marinate the steaks and keep aside for 30-40 minutes.
2. Grill the steaks for 5-6 minutes per side. Remove, then cool before slicing. Serve.

NUTRITION:

Calories: 473; Fat: 17.6g; Protein: 60.8g; Carbohydrates: 1.6g.

WEDNESDAY - DAY 24 - DINNER
TURKISH STYLE BELL PEPPERS

Preparation Time: 15 minutes

Cooking Time: 50 minutes

Servings: 4

INGREDIENTS:

4 large organic eggs

½ cup plus 2 tablespoons Parmesan cheese, grated and divided

½ cup mozzarella cheese, shredded

½ cup ricotta cheese

1 teaspoon garlic powder

¼ teaspoon dried parsley

2 medium bell peppers, cut in half and seeded

¼ cup fresh baby spinach leaves

DIRECTIONS:

1. Preheat the oven to 375°F and lightly, grease a baking dish.
2. In a small food processor, place the eggs, ½ cup of Parmesan, mozzarella, ricotta cheese, garlic powder and parsley and pulse until well combined.
3. Arrange the bell pepper halves into prepared baking dish, cut side up.
4. Place the cheese mixture into each pepper half and top each with a few spinach leaves.
5. With a fork, push the spinach leaves into the cheese mixture.
6. With a piece of foil, cover the baking dish and bake for about 35-45 minutes.
7. Now, set the oven to broiler on high.
8. Top each bell pepper half with the remaining Parmesan cheese and broil for about 3-5 minutes.
9. Remove from the oven and serve hot.

NUTRITION:

Calories: 191; Fat: 11.2g; Protein: 16.6g; Carbohydrates: 7g.

THURSDAY - DAY 25 - BREAKFAST

BERRY SOY YOGURT PARFAIT

Preparation Time: 2-4 minutes

Cooking Time: 0 minutes

Servings: 1

INGREDIENTS:

One carton vanilla cultured soy yogurt

¼ cup granola (gluten-free)

1 cup berries (you can take strawberries, blueberries, raspberries, blackberries)

DIRECTIONS:

1. Put half of the yogurt in a glass jar or serving dish.
2. On the top put half of the berries.
3. Then sprinkle with half of granola
4. Repeat layers.

NUTRITION:

Calories: 244; Fat: 3.1g; Protein: 1.4g; Carbohydrates: 11.3g.

THURSDAY - DAY 25 - LUNCH
SESAME CHICKEN SALAD

Preparation Time: 20 minutes

Cooking Time: 0 minutes

Servings: 4

INGREDIENTS:

1 tablespoon sesame seeds

1 cucumber, peeled, halved lengthwise, and sliced.

3.5 ounces cabbage, chopped

2 ounces pak choi, finely chopped

½ red onion, thinly sliced

0.7-ounce large parsley, chopped

5 ounces cooked chicken, minced

For the dressing:

1 tablespoon extra virgin olive oil

1 teaspoon sesame oil

1 lime juice

1 teaspoon light honey

2 teaspoons soy sauce

DIRECTIONS:

1. Roast your sesame seeds in a dry pan for 2 minutes until they become slightly golden and fragrant.
2. Transfer to a plate to cool.
3. In a small bowl, mix olive oil, sesame oil, lime juice, honey, and soy sauce to prepare the dressing.
4. Place the cucumber, black cabbage, pak-choi, red onion, and parsley in a large bowl and mix gently.
5. Pour over the dressing and mix again.
6. Distribute the salad between two dishes and complete with the shredded chicken. Sprinkle with sesame seeds just before serving.

NUTRITION:

Calories: 345; Fat: 5g; Protein: 4g; Carbohydrates: 10g.

THURSDAY - DAY 25 - DINNER

BUTTERED SALMON

Preparation Time: 10 minutes

Cooking Time: 10 minutes

Servings: 4

INGREDIENTS:

4 (5-ounce) skin-on, boneless salmon fillets

Salt and ground black pepper, to taste

1 tablespoon olive oil

3 tablespoons butter

2 tablespoons lemon juice

2 tablespoons fresh rosemary, minced

1 teaspoon lemon zest, grated

DIRECTIONS:

1. Season the salmon fillets with salt and black pepper evenly.
2. In a non-stick wok, heat oil over medium heat.
3. Place the salmon fillets, skin side down, and cook for about 3-5 minutes, without stirring.
4. Flip the salmon fillets and cook for about 2 minutes.
5. Add the butter, lemon juice, rosemary, and lemon zest, and cook for about 2 minutes, spooning the butter sauce over the salmon fillets occasionally.
6. Serve hot.

NUTRITION:

Calories: 301; Fat: 21.2g; Protein: 27.7g; Carbohydrates: 1.3g.

FRIDAY - DAY 26 - BREAKFAST

CHEESECAKE CUPS

Preparation Time: 5 minutes

Cooking Time: 0 minutes

Servings: 4 servings

INGREDIENTS:

8 ounces cream cheese, softened

2 ounces heavy cream

1 teaspoon Stevia Glycerite

1 teaspoon Splenda

1 teaspoon vanilla flavoring (Frontier Organic)

DIRECTIONS:

1. Combine all the ingredients.
2. Whip until a pudding consistency is achieved.
3. Divide into cups.
4. Refrigerate until served!

NUTRITION:

Calories: 205; Fat: 19g; Protein: 5g; Carbohydrates: 2g.

FRIDAY - DAY 26 - LUNCH
TUNA CAKES

Preparation Time: 15 minutes

Cooking Time: 10 minutes

Servings: 2

INGREDIENTS:

1 (15-ounce) can water-packed tuna, drained

½ celery stalk, chopped

2 tablespoons fresh parsley, chopped

1 teaspoon fresh dill, chopped

2 tablespoons walnuts, chopped

2 tablespoons mayonnaise

1 organic egg, beaten

1 tablespoon butter

3 cups lettuce

DIRECTIONS:

1. Add all ingredients (except the butter and lettuce) in a bowl and mix until well-combined.
2. Make two equal-sized patties from the mixture.
3. Melt some butter and cook the patties for about 2-3 minutes.
4. Carefully flip the side and cook for about 2-3 minutes.
5. Divide the lettuce onto serving plates.
6. Top each plate with one burger and serve.

NUTRITION:

Calories: 267; Fat: 12.5g; Protein: 11.5g; Carbohydrates: 3.8g.

FRIDAY - DAY 26 - DINNER

GREEK VEGGIE BRIAM

Preparation Time: 10 minutes

Cooking Time: 30 minutes

Servings: 4

INGREDIENTS:

1/3 cup good-quality olive oil, divided

1 onion, thinly sliced

1 tablespoon minced garlic

¾ small eggplant, diced

2 zucchinis, diced

2 cups chopped cauliflower

1 red bell pepper, diced

2 cups diced tomatoes

2 tablespoons chopped fresh parsley

2 tablespoons chopped fresh oregano

Sea salt, for seasoning

Freshly ground black pepper, for seasoning

1 ½ cups crumbled feta cheese

¼ cup pumpkin seeds

DIRECTIONS:

1. Preheat the oven. Set the oven to broil and lightly grease a 9- by-13-inch casserole dish with olive oil.
2. Sauté the aromatics in a medium stockpot over medium heat, warm 3 tablespoons of the olive oil. Add the onion and garlic and sauté until they've softened, about 3 minutes.
3. Sauté the vegetables. Stir in the eggplant, cook, stirring occasionally.
4. Add the zucchini, cauliflower, and red bell pepper and cook for 5 minutes.
5. Stir in the tomatoes, parsley, and oregano and cook, stirring from time to time, until the vegetables are tender, about 10 minutes. Season it with salt and pepper.
6. Broil. Put vegetable mix in the casserole dish and top with the crumbled feta. Broil until the cheese is melted.
7. Serve. Divide the casserole between four plates and top it with the pumpkin seeds. Drizzle with the remaining olive oil.

NUTRITION:

Calories: 341; Fat: 5.1g; Protein: 1.4g; Carbohydrates: 1.2g.

SATURDAY - DAY 27 - BREAKFAST

STRAWBERRY SHAKE

Preparation Time: 5 minutes

Cooking Time: 0 minutes

Servings: 1 serving

INGREDIENTS:

¾ cup coconut milk (from the carton)

¼ cup heavy cream

7 ice cubes

2 tablespoons sugar-free strawberry

Torani syrup

¼ teaspoon Xanthan Gum

DIRECTIONS:

1. Combine all the ingredients into blender.
2. Blend for 1-2 minutes.
3. Serve!

NUTRITION:

Calories: 270; Fat: 27g; Protein: 2.5g; Carbohydrates: 6.5g.

SATURDAY - DAY 27 - LUNCH

PIZZA BIANCA

Preparation Time: 10 minutes

Cooking Time: 10 minutes

Servings: 2

INGREDIENTS:

2 tablespoons olive oil

4 eggs

2 tablespoons water

1 jalapeño pepper, diced

¼ cup mozzarella cheese, shredded

2 chives, chopped

2 cups egg Alfredo sauce

½ teaspoon oregano

½ cup mushrooms, sliced

DIRECTIONS:

1. Preheat oven to 360°F.
2. In a bowl, whisk eggs, water, and oregano. Heat the olive oil in a large skillet.
3. The egg mixture must be poured in, then let it cook until set, flipping once.
4. Remove and spread the Alfredo sauce and jalapeño pepper all over.
5. Top with mozzarella cheese, mushrooms and chives. Let it bake for 10 minutes

NUTRITION:

Calories: 314; Fat: 15.6g; Protein: 10.4g; Carbohydrates: 5.9g.

SATURDAY - DAY 27 - DINNER

ROASTED TENDERLOIN

Preparation Time: 10 minutes

Cooking Time: 50 minutes

Servings: 10

INGREDIENTS:

1 grass-fed beef tenderloin roast

4 garlic cloves

1 tablespoon rosemary

Salt

Ground black pepper

1 tablespoon olive oil

DIRECTIONS:

1. Warm-up oven to 425°F.
2. Place beef meat into the prepared roasting pan. Massage with garlic, rosemary, salt, and black pepper and oil. Roast the beef for 45-50 minutes.
3. Remove, cool, slice, and serve.

NUTRITION:

Calories: 295; Fat: 13.9g; Protein: 39.5g; Carbohydrates: 0.6g.

SUNDAY - DAY 28 - BREAKFAST

BACON HASH

Preparation Time: 5 minutes

Cooking Time: 10 minutes

Servings: 2

INGREDIENTS:

1 small green pepper

2 jalapeno peppers

1 small onion

4 eggs

6 bacon slices

DIRECTIONS:

1. Chop the bacon into chunks using a food processor. Set aside for now. Slice the onions and peppers into thin strips. Dice the jalapenos as small as possible.
2. Heat a skillet and fry the veggies. Once browned, combine the ingredients and cook until crispy. Place on a serving dish with fried eggs.

NUTRITION:

Calories: 366; Fat: 24g; Protein: 23g; Carbohydrates: 9g.

SUNDAY - DAY 28 - LUNCH

TEMPURA ZUCCHINI WITH CREAM CHEESE DIP

Preparation Time: 15 minutes

Cooking Time: 15 minutes

Servings: 4

INGREDIENTS:

Tempura zucchinis:

1 ½ cups (200g) almond flour

2 tablespoons heavy cream

1 teaspoon salt

2 tablespoons olive oil + extra for frying

1 ¼ cups (300ml) water

½ tablespoon sugar-free maple syrup

2 large zucchinis, cut into 1-inch thick strips

Cream cheese dip:

8 onces cream cheese, room temperature

½ cup (113g) sour cream

1 teaspoon taco seasoning

1 scallion, chopped

1 green chili, deseeded and minced

DIRECTIONS:

1. In a bowl, mix the almond flour, heavy cream, salt, peanut oil, water, and maple syrup.
2. Dredge the zucchini strips in the mixture until well-coated.
3. Heat about four tablespoons of olive oil in a non-stick skillet.
4. Working in batches, use tongs to remove the zucchinis (draining extra liquid) into the oil.
5. Fry per side for 1 to 2 minutes and remove the zucchinis onto a paper towel-lined plate to drain grease.
6. In a bowl or container, mix the cream cheese, taco seasoning, sour cream, scallion, and green chili.
7. Serve the tempura zucchinis with the cream cheese dip.

NUTRITION:

Calories: 316; Fat: 8.4g; Protein: 5.1g; Carbohydrates: 4.1g.

SUNDAY - DAY 28 - DINNER

CREAMY PARMESAN SHRIMP

Preparation Time: 10 minutes

Cooking Time: 20 minutes

Servings: 4

INGREDIENTS:

1 ½ pounds shrimp

½ cup chicken stock

¼ teaspoon red pepper flakes

1 cup parmesan cheese, grated

1 cup fresh basil leaves

1 ½ cups heavy cream

¼ teaspoon paprika

3 ounces roasted red peppers, sliced

½ onion, minced

1 tablespoon garlic, minced

3 tablespoons butter

Pepper to taste

Salt to taste

DIRECTIONS:

1. Melt 2 tablespoons butter in a pan over medium heat.
2. Season shrimp with pepper and salt and sear in a pan for 1-2 minutes. Transfer shrimp on a plate.
3. Add remaining butter in a pan.
4. Add red chili flakes, paprika, roasted peppers, garlic, onion, pepper, and salt and cook for 5 minutes.
5. Add stock and stir well and cook until liquid reduced by half.
6. Turn heat to low, add cream and stir for 1-2 minutes.
7. Add basil and parmesan cheese and stir for 1-2 minutes.
8. Return shrimp to the pan and cook for 1-2 minutes.
9. Serve and enjoy.

NUTRITION:

Calories: 524; Fat: 33.2g; Protein: 47.8g; Carbohydrates: 8.3g.

Measurement and Conversions

CUPS	OZ	G	TBSP	TSP	ML
1	8	225	16	48	250
3/4	6	170	12	36	175
2/3	5	140	11	32	150
1/2	4	115	8	24	125
1/3	3	70	5	16	70
1/4	2	60	4	12	60
1/8	1	30	2	6	30
1/16	1/2	15	1	3	15

250°F	300°F	325°F	350°F	400°F	450°F
120°C	150°F	160°C	175°C	200°C	230°C

About the Author

Carleigh Johnson is a registered dietitian, and a licensed dietitian. She has been a practicing dietitian for over 10 years. Lola is passionate about empowering people to lead active healthy lifestyles by teaching them the personalized skills they need to fuel themselves with whole foods while maintaining a healthy life balance.

Made in the USA
Monee, IL
31 March 2025

14921949R10059